THE GENTLE ART OF

Yoga

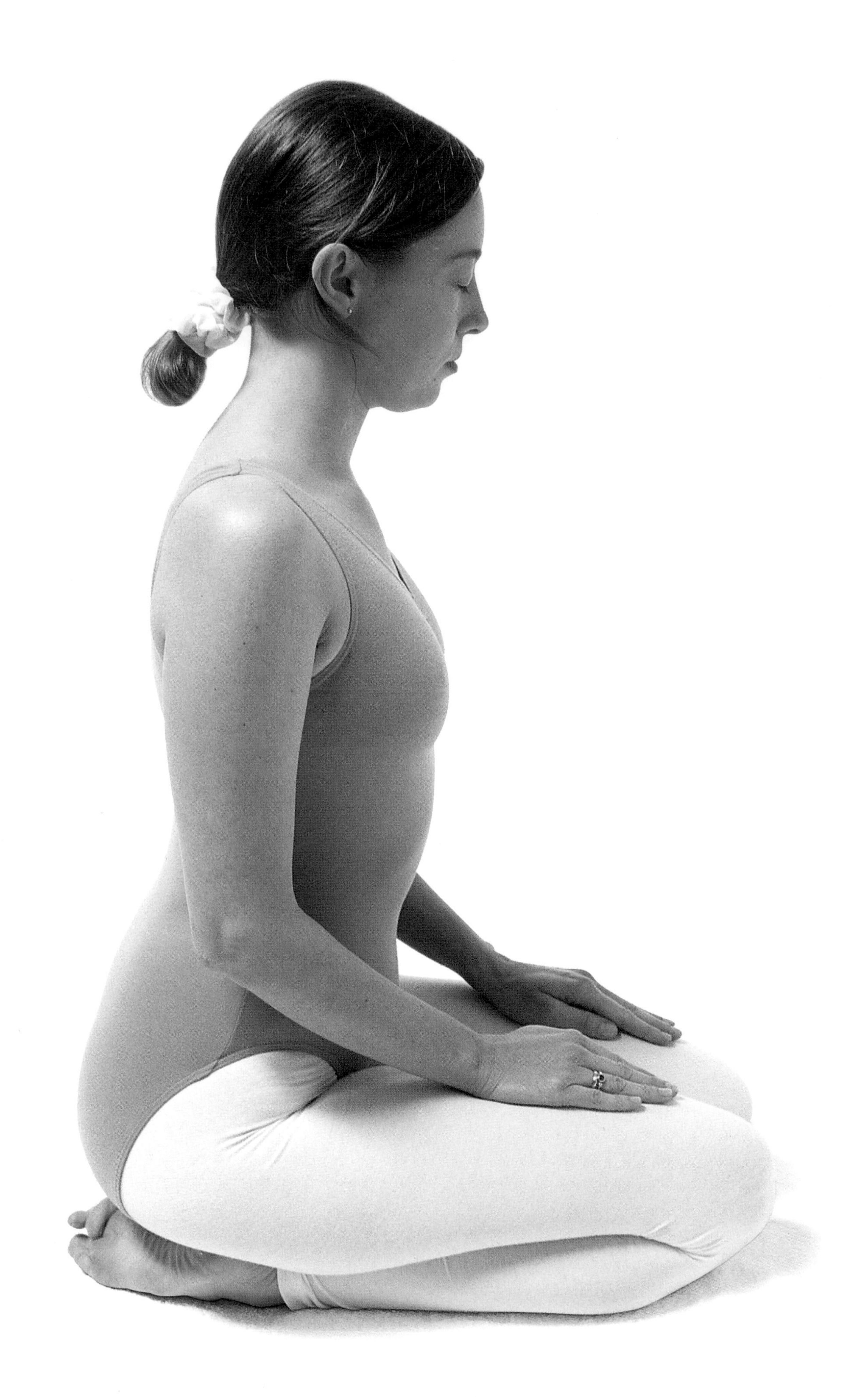

THE GENTLE ART OF

Yoga

CHANCELLOR
PRESS

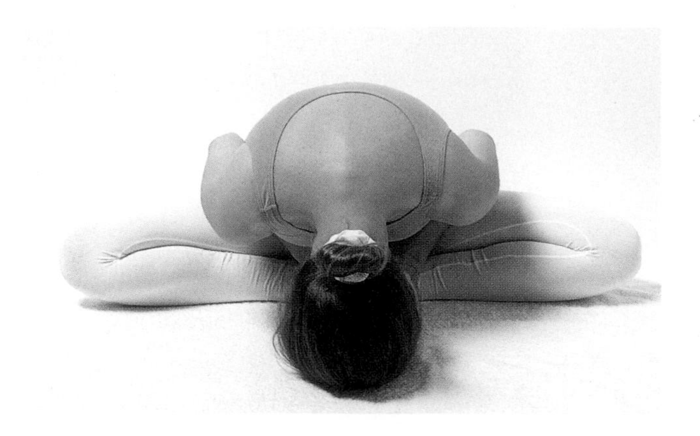

Contents

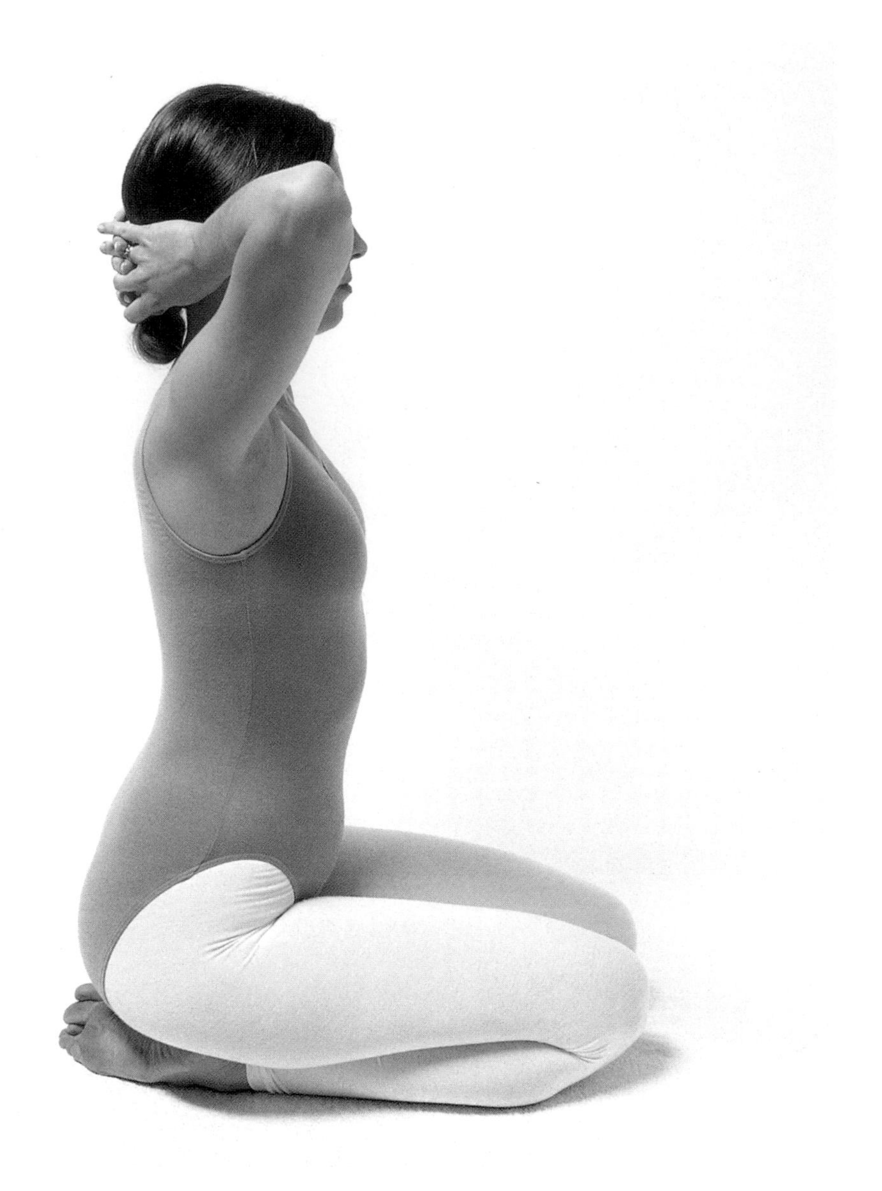

How to Use This Book

This book is intended to provide a short introductory course for the beginner yoga student. It is suitable for those with little or no previous yoga experience.

The practices in this book are described in simple, step-by-step instructions, with accompanying photographs. Highlighted or boxed text will emphasize any information to which you need pay particular attention.

The layout enables you to progress through the book from beginning to end in a logical and harmonious sequence. It is recommended you work through the whole book, at least once, as this will give you a true understanding of a total yoga practice. Once you have done this, you may like to concentrate on one section at a time.

The major aim of this book is to introduce yoga in a manner which is gentle, relaxing, non-threatening and, most importantly, enjoyable.

The Art of Yoga

Yoga brings harmony to our existence.
A gentle exercise, yoga is also a philosophy,
a health system and a way of life.

Yoga, although now very popular in the Western world, still remains something of an enigma. Most people have heard of yoga. They might have seen brochures or read articles; and many people have attended classes. Yet there is still confusion as to what yoga really is.

A common misconception is that yoga is a mystical form of exercise during which you contort the body into a series of bizarre positions. Many people imagine strange rituals and torturing work-outs. None of these things is true. Yoga is a simple and gentle activity, suitable for everyone. The practice of yoga is not a religion.

The word yoga comes from the Sanskrit root word "yuj" which means to yoke or to bind. This is the essence of yoga — to unify the physical body with the mind and with the vital energy flowing within. When these components move closer together, one experiences a sense of harmony and balance. In the modern world, life is busy and it is common to feel fragmented or displaced. Yoga helps to re-connect the fragments and bring a stillness to personal existence.

Yoga also works on all aspects of health to encourage a strong body, a sharp mind, and the ability to reduce the effects of stress. As you practice yoga, notice how the worries of the day dissolve and how life itself begins to flow more easily.

What does yoga involve?

The practice of yoga involves a number of easy techniques which work together to bring about health and tranquillity.

These techniques include:

- physical postures (asanas) — the basis of yoga, asanas work gently to increase flexibility, strengthen the muscles and tone all body systems.
- breathing exercises (pranayama) — these techniques help to increase energy levels, calm the emotions and sharpen the mind.
- meditation (dhyana) — brings a quietness to the whole being and offers a personal refuge from internal and external stresses.
- total relaxation (yoga nidra) — a deep relaxation of the body and mind which soothes and rejuvenates.

All these aspects of yoga practice act together to nurture the whole being. Yoga is a non-competitive activity, a gentle art. There is no puffing, no panting, no strain and no pain. Remember to respect your body, work at your own pace, and simply enjoy your yoga as precious time away from daily cares.

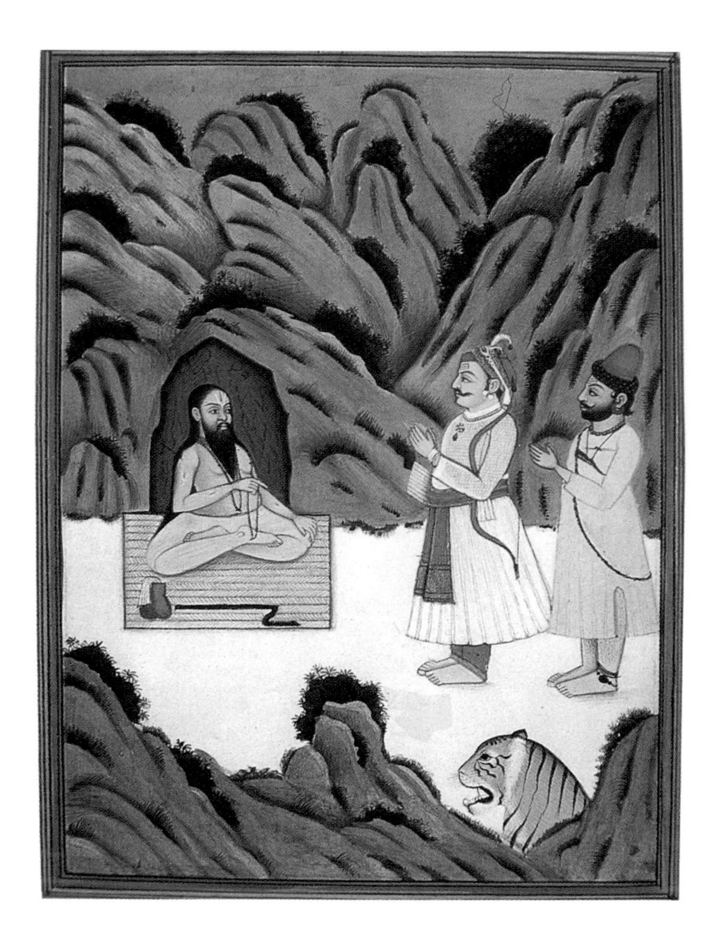

Yoga was first developed as a philosophy of life; the practices then developed to sustain this philosophy. Yoga emphasizes the necessity of harmony with the whole.

The history of yoga

The practice of yoga is thousands of years old. It was in ancient times that human beings first began to explore ways of illuminating and understanding their own existence. Before the written word, all important knowledge was passed down in the form of stories, fables and artwork. In this way, information was accumulated and cultures developed. This was how the philosophy and practice of yoga came into being. In the Indus Valley archaeologists have found carvings and sculptures depicting yoga practices. They were created by the highly civilized community which flourished in this area, now part of Pakistan, between 2000 and 1000 BC.

Several major works on the philosophy and practice of yoga were compiled throughout India's history. As peoples of Asia moved across the continent and into India, a rich and complex culture was developed. Yoga was first developed as a philosophy of life; the practices were developed to sustain this philosophy. The major teachings are:

The Vedas

About two thousand years BC the Aryan race began to migrate into India from Iran. The *Vedas* are the teachings of the Aryans and are believed to be the basis of the Hindu religion. The *Vedas* consist of four books of hymns, the best known being the *Rig-Veda*. The hymns stress the omnipotent power of nature. It is this regard for natural principles which is the essence of yoga.

The Upanishads

These philosophical writings probably composed between 800 and 200 BC address the issue of spiritual enlightenment. The practice of yoga and meditation is first alluded to in the *Upanishads*. Its teachings espouse the importance of finding "stillness" in life and stability in the senses.

Bhagavad Gita

The *Bhagavad Gita* is a classic text, written about 300 BC. Written as a spiritual poem, it is part of a larger Sanskrit epic called the *Mahabharata*. It speaks of three paths as the basis of life: Jnana yoga (knowledge), Bhakti yoga (devotion) and Karma yoga (action). The *Bhagavad Gita* is translated into English and is readily available.

Yoga Sutras

Patanjali, a Hindu sage, was the first to rationalize and commit to writing the basic philosophies of yoga practice. He did this in eight concise aphorisms or small paragraphs. These aphorisms, thought to be written between 200 BC and 300 AD, are easy to comprehend. They offer a set of eight practices and principles for a healthy, contented life. The eight limbs to yoga practice are:

1. Yama: moral codes of a universal nature
2. Niyama: personal conduct
3. Asanas: the practice of postures
4. Pranayama: breath control
5. Pratyahara: control of the senses
6. Dharana: the power of concentration
7. Dhyana: the stillness of meditation
8. Samadhi: contemplation and reflection

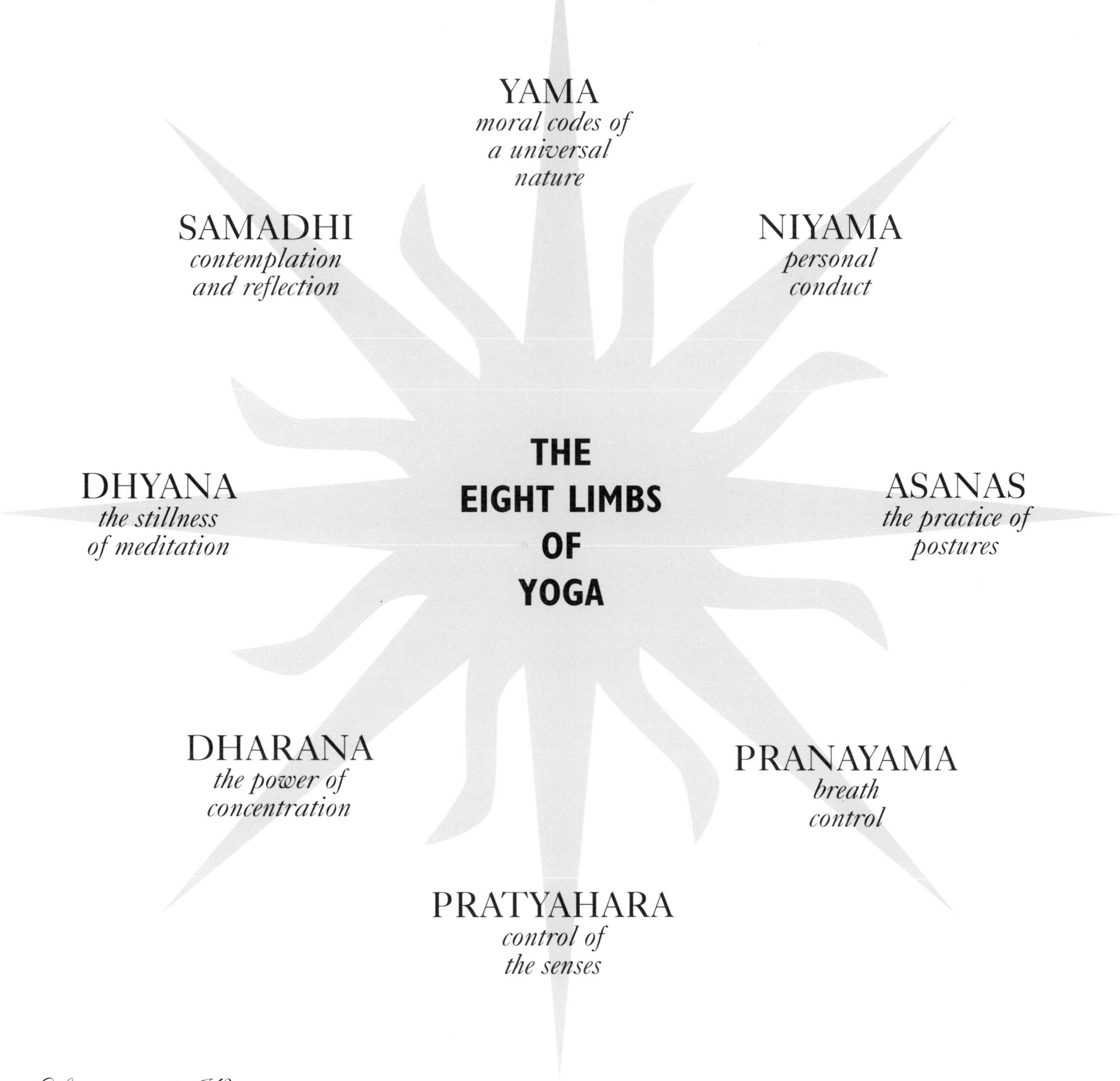

YAMA
moral codes of a universal nature

SAMADHI
contemplation and reflection

NIYAMA
personal conduct

THE EIGHT LIMBS OF YOGA

DHYANA
the stillness of meditation

ASANAS
the practice of postures

DHARANA
the power of concentration

PRANAYAMA
breath control

PRATYAHARA
control of the senses

Yoga in the West

Yoga was first introduced to the Western world as a result of the process of colonization of India during the 18th and 19th centuries. Travel to the East became popular in the 19th century and an interest in exotic cultures grew. Indian teachers of yoga traveled west and ancient texts were translated.

This interest has continued into the 20th century. The "alternative" era of the 1960s and 1970s saw this enthusiasm in yoga escalate.

Today yoga is very popular in the West. In most cities and towns, yoga classes are available. The gentle exercise, the relaxation, and refuge from daily stress prove yoga to be an ideal pastime for the modern world.

Yoga is an ancient philosophy, but it has stood the test of time and is appropriate for any person, in any place, and any era.

Yoga and health

One of the original holistic health systems, the practice of yoga is among the simplest ways to achieve and maintain perfect health. It is a gentle system, which addresses every part of one's being.

Yoga works because it balances the health on three levels: the physical body, the mental sphere and the vital energy. In this way all contributing factors to ill-health are treated and harmony resides again. Remember, health is a natural state. Illness is not.

The practice of yoga fosters respect for your body and for your health.

Regular yoga practice helps us deal with daily stress, anxiety, pain or grief. A sense of objectivity is developed, so we can learn to stand apart and address life's situations. Yoga strengthens inner resilience.

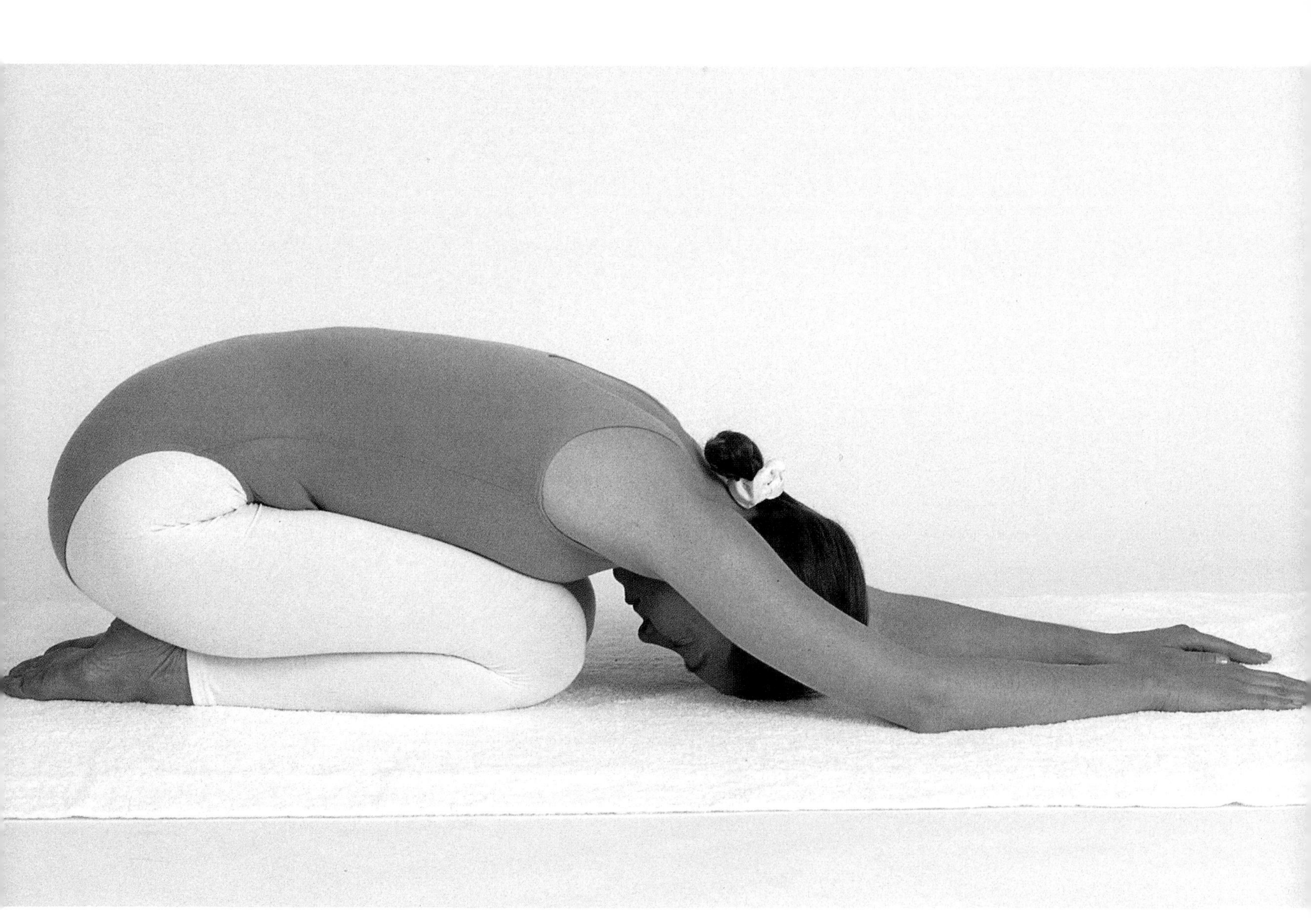

THE GENERAL BENEFITS OF YOGA

Physical body

- *strengthens and tones the muscles*
- *improves flexibility*
- *encourages grace of movement*
- *corrects poor posture*
- *aligns the spine*
- *stimulates and balances the body systems: cardiovascular/respiratory/endocrine/digestive/urinary/reproductive/lymphatic*

(see feature, "An overview of the body", page 12)

- *massages all the abdominal organs*
- *removes toxins from the body*

With each yoga posture, the organs, the muscles and the skeletal frame are nourished by a fresh supply of blood carrying nutrition and oxygen. Every cell of the body is enlivened.

Mental sphere

- *promotes relaxation*
- *calms and stills the mind*
- *sharpens the thought processes*
- *encourages clarity and concentration*
- *soothes the emotions and balances the moods*

Regular yoga practice helps us deal with daily stress, anxiety, pain or grief. A sense of objectivity is developed, so we can learn to stand apart and address life's situations. Yoga strengthens inner resilience.

Vital energy

- *unblocks stagnant energy*
- *stimulates a flow of vibrant energy throughout the body's systems*
- *redirects energy to all parts of the body*

Tiredness and fatigue are common complaints of the modern world. Yoga helps rid the body of stale energy and awaken new vitality.

Yoga and a healthy lifestyle

The body is affected by everything inside us and around us. This includes what we eat, what we breathe, what we do, what we think and how we feel. There is no need to live like a monk — moderation in all things is the key. However, you will find the more you practice yoga, the more you will lean towards a healthy lifestyle.

The benefits of yoga will be greatly enhanced by incorporating:

- a healthy, balanced diet
- plenty of pure water
- fresh air
- some sunshine
- adequate, but not too much, sleep
- good hygiene
- a balance of physical and mental activity
- a balance of work and play.

Yoga as a treatment

Yoga practice complements all other types of health care. Whether the chosen treatment is modern medicine or one of the array of "alternative" health systems, yoga can be safely incorporated into the treatment routine. Yoga encourages self healing, strength of body and clarity of mind. This can only boost the healing process.

Regular yoga practice can be beneficial to a number of specific illnesses. It has been used as a complete treatment regime by many people. Often illnesses can be alleviated, regardless of whether the condition is acute or long-standing.

However, always consult your health practitioner before beginning yoga practice for the first time, and consult a yoga teacher to advise on specific postures for your condition. Not all postures are suitable for everyone.

There are some illnesses which should be approached with special care. (See 'Caution' on page 15).

An overview of the body

The human body is a complex and intriguing structure. It is made up of many intricate parts which work together in complete unison. Health begins to decline when this harmony is unbalanced.

The brain and the spine make up the central nervous system. The brain is connected to the spine, and the spine to a network of nerves called the peripheral nervous system.

The peripheral nervous system relays information to the brain, via the spine, about the state of the body and the external environment. In return the brain informs the body which then reacts in an appropriate way. As mediator in this exchange, it is essential the spine is kept healthy and strong.

With each yoga posture, the organs, the muscles and the skeletal frame are nourished by a fresh supply of blood carrying nutrition and oxygen. Every cell of the body is enlivened.

The body also runs a number of other systems, each with their own functions:

- cardiovascular system – veins and arteries which carry blood to the heart and around the body providing the system with nutrition and oxygen
- respiratory system – takes oxygen into the body and expels carbon dioxide
- endocrine system– is made up of hormone-producing glands which control the internal environment of the body
- digestive system – provides energy to the body from the food we eat, and disposes of any waste matter
- urinary system – regulates the salts in the body and eliminates toxins via urine output
- reproductive system – controls sexual and reproductive functioning
- lymphatic (immune) system – protects the body against invading organisms and encourages resistance to disease

The muscles and the skeleton physically hold the whole structure together. Skin and hair protect the body. Sensory organs such as the eyes, ears, nose and tongue perceive the world around us. The emotions and thoughts are also a major contributor to overall health.

As well, there is the vital energy which flows through every cell, every structure. You cannot see it, but you can feel whether it is flowing strongly or weakly at any given time.

There is not any part of the body which is not intrinsically connected to the whole. In order for your body to work well, every component must be functioning smoothly.

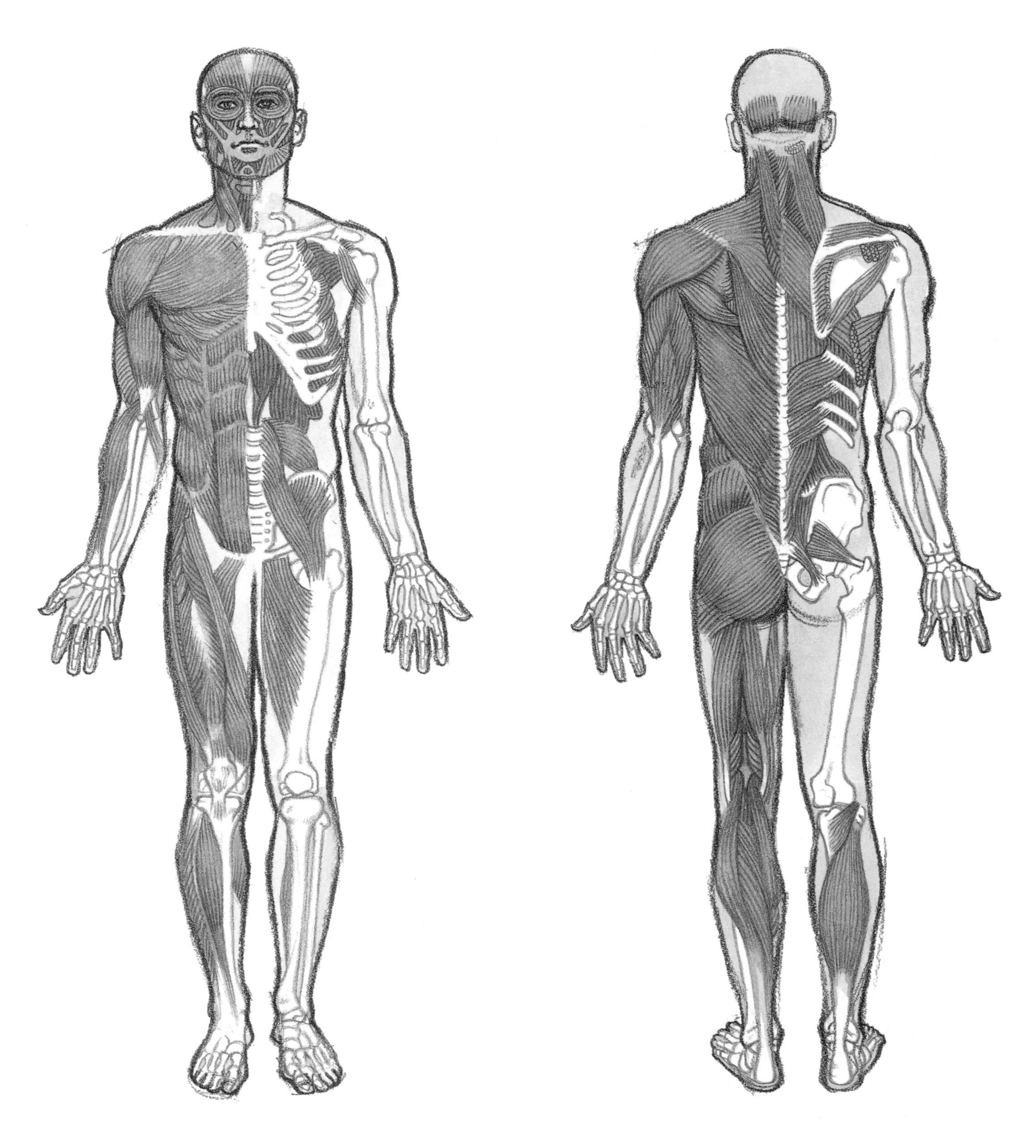

Muscular system — front view

Muscular system — back view

Is yoga for you?

With few exceptions, everyone can practice yoga. Yoga is suitable for people at all levels of fitness and all body shapes. It is equally suited to men and women, and people of all ages will benefit. It is the perfect activity to practice throughout a lifetime.

Children love yoga and tend to learn the postures without effort. As many of the poses imitate animals, children view them as fun. The calming attributes of yoga practice make it especially therapeutic for hyperactive children. The postures will also help the child develop a healthy body and good posture.

Yoga soothes the torments of teenage years and helps the adult with the battles of life. In old age, yoga is an indispensable tool for maintaining a finely tuned body and mind.

Yoga is non-competitive and everyone is free to work at their own pace. There is no pressure or strain. There is no need for self-consciousness. Yoga is for everyone to enjoy.

Yoga classes

There are now many yoga classes available should you want the guidance of a teacher. You may have noticed different types of yoga advertised, for example:

- Hatha yoga – This is a general term which refers to the practice of yoga postures. Most beginners' hatha classes concentrate on gentle poses and include a relaxation session;
- Iyengar yoga – This is hatha yoga as adopted for the Western world by B.K.S Iyengar. These classes focus on a large spectrum of postures which strengthen and maintain the body;
- Raja yoga – mostly meditative practices.

Depending on the teacher and the style of yoga, some classes concentrate more on postures, while others incorporate breathing, meditation and relaxation techniques. The best way to find the ideal class for your own needs is to ask the teacher for a general description of the class content. Sample a number of classes, and see which you prefer.

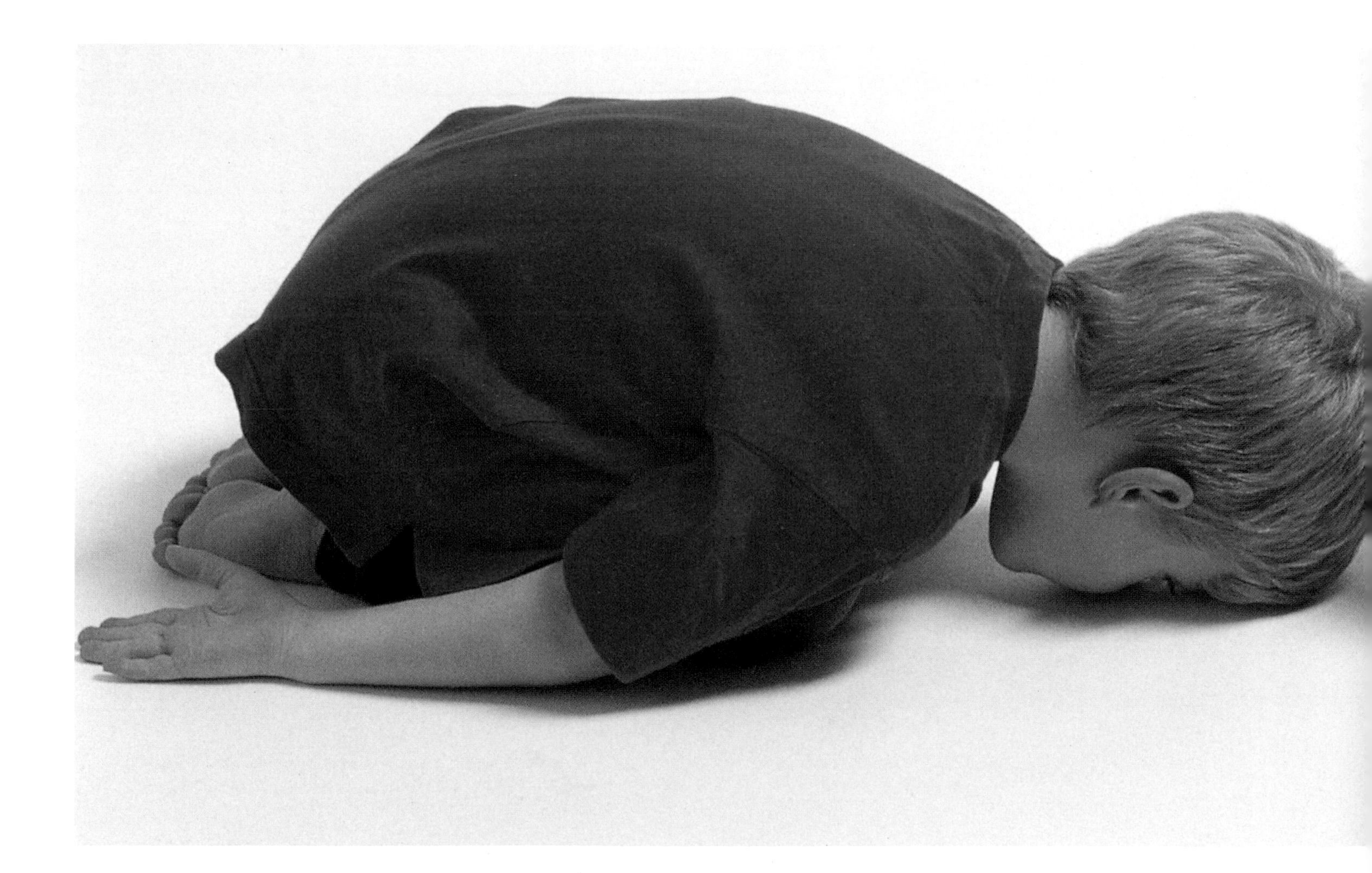

Yoga and menstruation

There are many postures which are not recommended during menstruation. At this time, the temperature of the body is raised. Some women may be experiencing pain or generally feeling unwell. Concentrate on cooling and calming postures, for example, rests and gentle stretches.

Avoid inverted and bending postures. See 'Sequences' on page 63, for a recommended schedule.

Yoga and pregnancy

Yoga can be of great benefit physically and emotionally to the expectant and new mother. There are many postures and breathing techniques which will ease the birth process and help maintain vitality after the birth. However, it is essential that you consult a health practitioner and a yoga teacher before attempting any postures during pregnancy. The best option is to attend special pre-natal yoga classes. Always avoid any postures which constrict the abdomen.

CAUTION

Before commencing yoga practice, it is advisable to consult a health practitioner if you have any of the following conditions:

- high blood pressure
- heart problems
- vertigo
- cancer/tumor
- diabetes
- HIV/AIDS
- Multiple Sclerosis
- ulcer
- hernia
- eye or ear problems
- any long term illness
- a recent operation

If you do have any of the above conditions, it does not mean you are excluded from practicing yoga. A carefully planned program will be both safe and therapeutic. It is important to know which postures to avoid — consult a teacher.

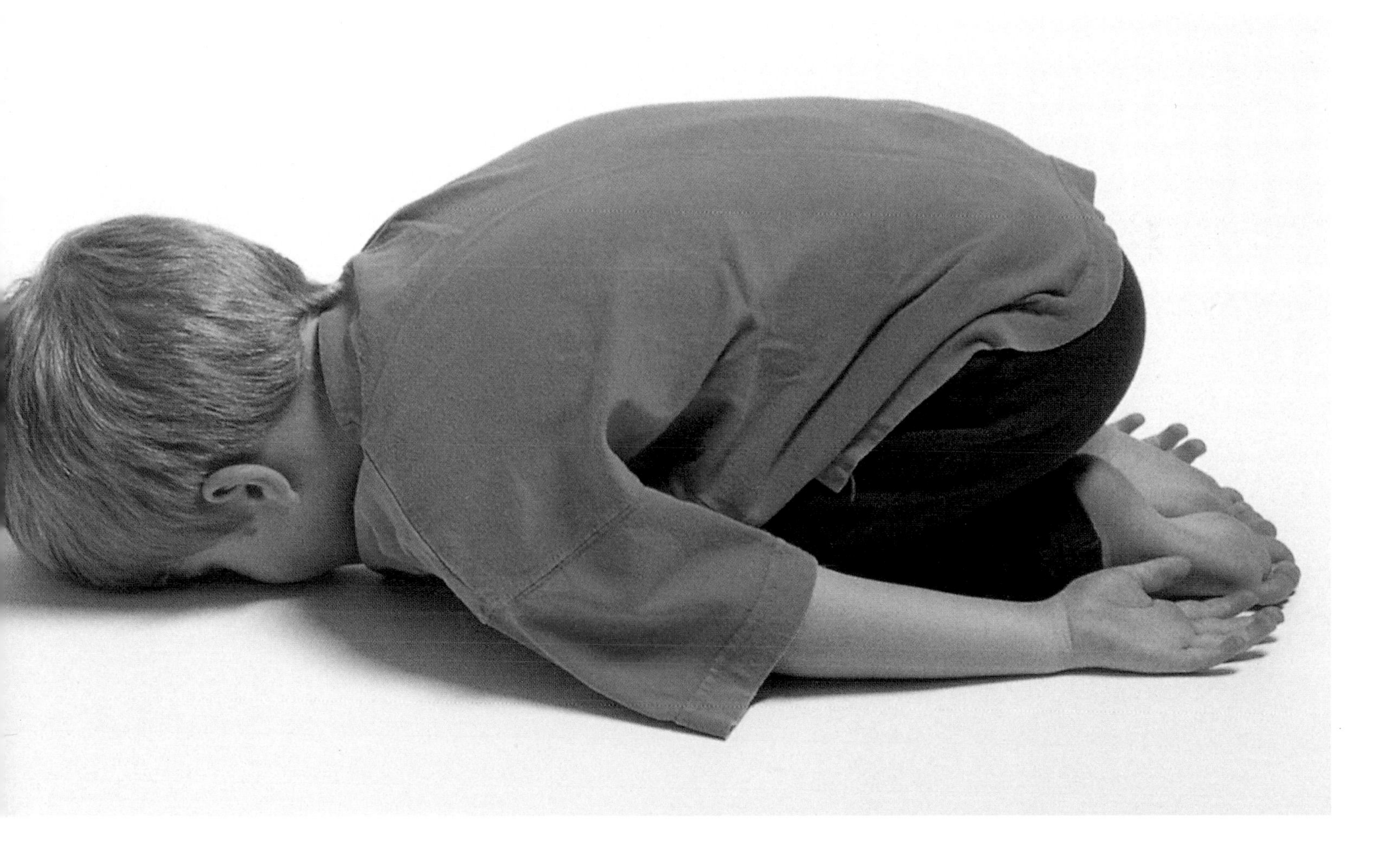

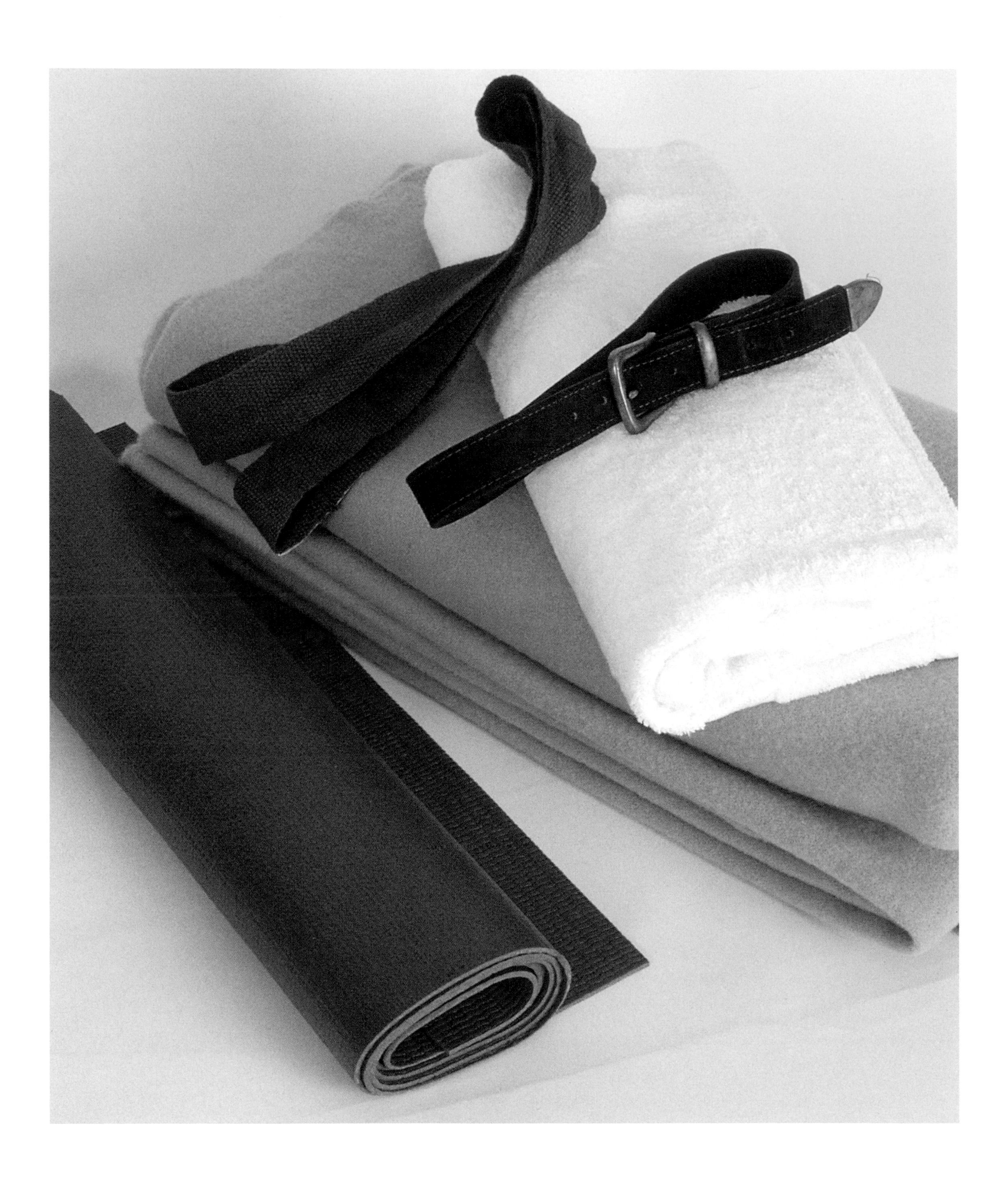

Preparation

Environment

Although yoga can be practiced anywhere, it is preferable to have your own space set aside. Ideally, choose a room which is light and airy, where the atmosphere is fresh and free from dust. Minimal furniture will ensure you do not injure yourself bumping into things. The floor should be even and level.

Clear an area of wall space, as some postures use a wall for support. Make sure the room is not too hot or cold. If you turn on a heater or fan, be certain it is located somewhere safe and out of the way.

Your yoga room should be quiet and calm; a space you look forward to being in. If possible, try not to be disturbed during yoga practice. Choose a time when you can be reasonably sure you will not be distracted, and take the phone off the hook.

For added atmosphere you may like to light a candle, burn incense, or heat some essential oils.

Equipment

There are only a few pieces of equipment you will need.

• A mat – A thin mat is excellent for support during postures. It should not be soft or spongy. Yoga mats can be purchased from rubber stores. Camping mats are also suitable. If your room is carpeted, you can practice without a mat — just put down a clean towel.

• Blankets – One or two folded blankets will protect the spine and neck in inverted postures; a blanket is also useful to keep you warm during breathing exercises, meditation and relaxation.

• Towels – Folded towels beneath the buttocks encourage correct posture when you are first learning yoga. They also prevent undue strain. You can use one of the blankets instead of a towel, if it is not too thick.

• A belt – If in some postures you find your elbows slipping outwards or knees upwards, try securing them in position with a belt.

• A rope – The use of a rope will help to improve flexibility in the stretching postures. It will also encourage you to swivel from the hips. Wrap the rope around the legs and gently extend the stretch.

Yourself

• Remove accessories such as watches and jewellery.

• Tie long hair back as it becomes a nuisance in forward bending postures.

• Clothing – Choose light, comfortable clothing which does not restrict the abdomen. Loose pants and a T-shirt is suitable as are any of the assortment of exercise leotards and outfits available today. Have a pair of socks handy as the feet often feel the cold during breathing exercises, meditation and relaxation practices.

• Eating – Do not practice yoga on a full stomach. Preferably allow several hours to pass after a large meal or one hour after a light meal. If you need to eat before yoga, try something easy to digest such as some white rice.

• Drinking – Do not drink too much liquid before practicing — you will find the postures much more comfortable if the bladder is empty.

• Bathing – A shower before yoga practice will help to warm and prepare the muscles. A shower after the practice will soothe the body and rinse away any toxins which have risen to the surface of the skin.

• Sun – Avoid yoga practice if you have been in strong sunshine for some time. Wait till the body has cooled down.

WHEN TO PRACTICE YOGA

You can practice yoga at any time of the day. First thing in the morning, when the stomach is empty, is perfect. The air is fresh and the earth's energy is high.

Practicing after work or before retiring can be very beneficial to the body and mind. It is desirable to expel accumulated stress before bed. Several short sessions a day is ideal.

See 'Sequences' on page 61.

The Practice of Postures

ASANAS

Asanas are physical postures. Aim to create a state of absolute comfort, where the body is relaxed the emotions calm, and the mind still.

The asanas are the physical limb of yoga practice. The postures work gently and subtly to improve flexibility, tone the muscles and strengthen the skeletal system. All the physiological functions are balanced so they are operating at an optimum and in harmony with each other. Toxins are eliminated from the body.

The practice of asanas also influences the psyche. By concentrating on the posture only, you will find the mind becomes quiet and the emotions steady.

Within the posture or asana, the mind, the body and breath become one. All time merges into the moment, and you become aware of the connection and the oneness of all things.

Before trying any of the following asanas, it is important that you refer to the 'Caution' on page 15 and read Chapter Two, 'Preparation' on page 16.

Before you begin

Following are a number of key phrases which will help you with your yoga practice. Keep these in mind at all times.

Work at your own pace

Yoga is not a competitive activity. Whether practicing alone, with a friend or in a class, do not compare yourself with others. Pay attention to your own being. Be aware of what is right for your body at the present time. This may vary from day to day. There is no hurry, no pressure; and there is plenty of time to progress at your own speed. Respect, and work with, your body.

Appreciate the moment

Learn to live in the present. When you are practicing postures try to forget about the activities of the day, the past or your plans for the future. Enjoy being in the here and now. This is not easy, but once achieved, you will feel enlightened and refreshed.

Easing in

Always ease into a posture. Never force the pose so you experience pain or strain. Instead, find a comfortable position, and with every exhalation, let your body stretch and loosen a little more. This is a gradual, subtle process. Notice how the body is willing to loosen and unwind, if encouraged gently. Do not push beyond your limits.

Awareness

Practice yoga with your full attention. If you attempt the postures carelessly, without awareness, the benefits will be minimal. Notice how your body is feeling while you are doing the posture; observe how the body reacts after the posture.

Be aware of which parts feel relaxed or energized, which parts feel worked, which parts are experiencing pain or strain. How has your mind reacted? Experience the posture to the full.

Remember to breathe

This is very important — correct use of the breath greatly enhances the value of asanas. The general rule is to breathe in as the body is stretched and breathe out as the body is contracted. The text specifies when you should be breathing in (inhaling) or breathing out (exhaling) with each posture.

Unless instructed, do not hold the breath. Breathe through the nose and always be aware of the breath. Rest between postures, ensuring the breath has returned to normal before starting a new posture.

Check your alignment

In some postures it is important that the head is in line with the spine, or that the arms are parallel, or that the body is lying straight. Always be aware of the shape your body is forming. This is called "alignment". When first practicing, a mirror may help.

Slow and dynamic

Rhythmic movement is incorporated into some postures, for example, Rocking and Rolling (see page 42) and the Twisting Triangle (see page 32). You may choose to move slowly or dynamically, depending on how you are feeling.

A slow practice is calming. A dynamic practice is performed quickly with vigor and raises the energy. Always rest after a dynamic practice.

Some asanas, like the Shoulder Stand, are physically more demanding than other postures.

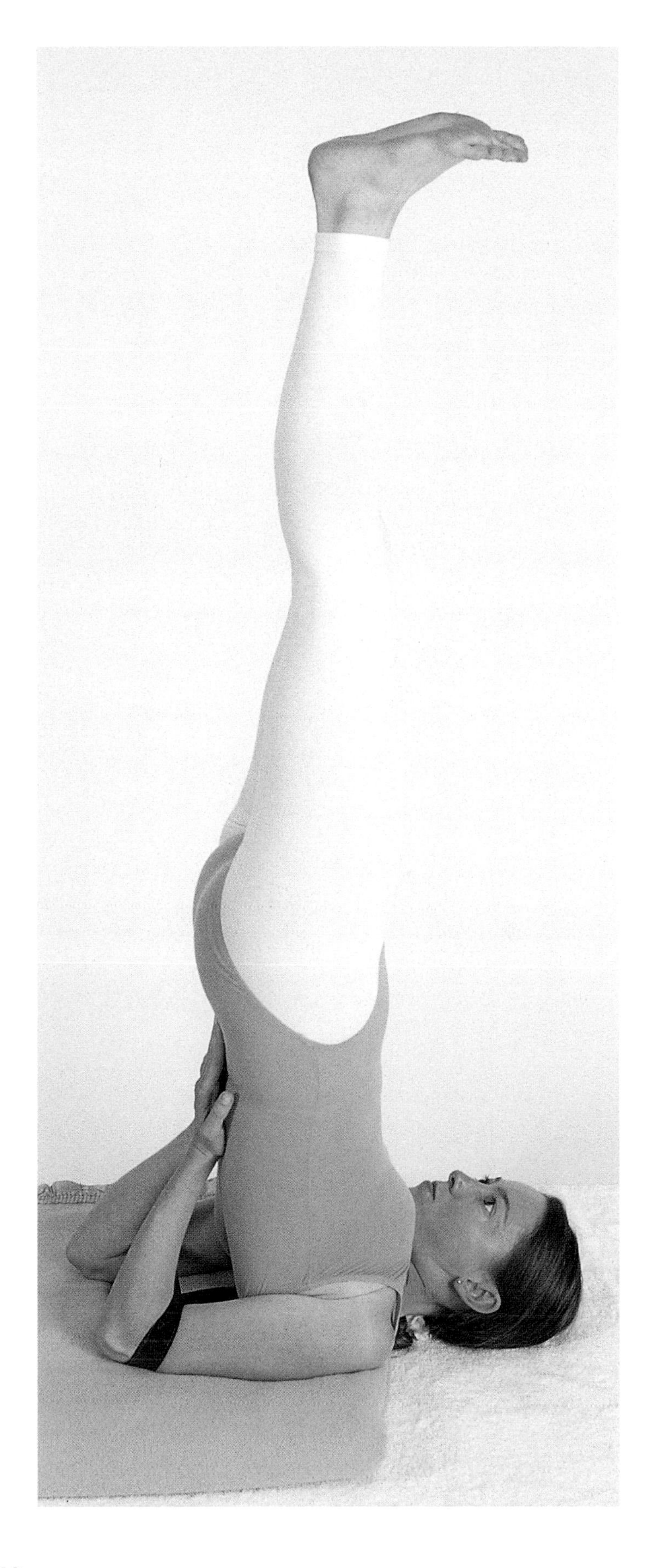

Classification of asanas

There is an endless range of asanas. Each has a unique nature. However, the asanas can be classified, and this helps our understanding of the practice of postures.

In this chapter we have divided the asanas into five sections: warm ups, standing postures, sitting postures, floor postures and inverted postures.

Warm ups are relaxing and prepare the joints for the yoga practice.

Within the other sections of this chapter, there is a classification code beside the title of each posture. This describes its general style and purpose. For example :

RESTS

Poses which calm and soothe the body. Use the rests between postures to rebalance and prepare for the next posture.

LOOSENERS

Help the body to gently unwind and activate energy within the body.

BALANCES

Encourage concentration and stillness of the mind, and develop grace and lightness.

STRETCHES

Elongate the muscles and improve flexibility.

BACKWARD BENDS

Strengthen the spine, open the chest, expel toxins and stimulate a fresh blood flow.

FORWARD BENDS

Massage abdominal organs, redirect blood to the brain and tone the back and leg muscles. Balance the body after backward bends.

TWISTS

Realign the spine, soothe muscles, stimulate the nervous system and adjust energy distribution.

INVERTED POSTURES

These poses reverse the force of gravity. They relieve tired legs, stimulate thyroid functioning, increase vitality and calm the emotions.

Each posture, or asana, should complement the last. A yoga session should flow easily from one posture to the next.

Many postures fit into more than one classification. A forward or backward bend is usually also a stretch. A twist may be a loosener. The classifications are only intended to provide an overview of the different types of postures and their benefits.

In yoga practice, each posture should complement the previous. A session should flow from one posture to the next easily and gently. The postures in this book have been arranged in this manner.

Try to include a range of postures in each yoga session. For an example see 'Sequences' on page 61. Remember to rest between postures. Your choice of postures and the number of times you repeat them will depend on how your body is feeling at the time. Listen to your body and experiment with different progressions.

Yoga is about balance and harmony — if you try a backward bend, always follow with a forward bend. If you stretch, curl up afterwards. Use this knowledge in daily life. If you carry a heavy bag, swap it from hand to hand.

As you work through the asanas, appreciate the harmony, not only within each posture, but within the total practice.

This is the art of yoga.

Warm-up exercises

Before beginning a yoga session, it is wise to perform a few warm-up exercises to help loosen and lubricate the joints. Early in the morning or after a day at the desk, muscles are often stiff and energy stagnant — use warm ups to awaken and refresh the whole body.

NECK ROLLS

1. Stand or sit in a comfortable position. Straighten your body and feel your head positioned directly above the spine. Very slowly and gently let your head drop so the chin is towards your chest. Notice the stretch at the base of the neck.

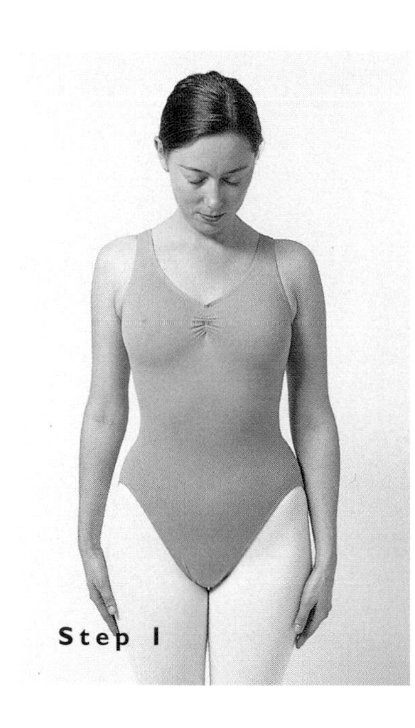
Step 1

2. Now let your head roll backwards gradually and look towards the ceiling. *Do not let your head fall back suddenly.* Repeat several times.

3. Return your head to the center position. Move your neck towards the right so the right ear is close to the right shoulder.

4. Now roll your head towards the left. Feel the muscles loosen and the vertebrae open, as you practice this exercise. Neck exercises are great tension releasers. Always treat your neck with care. It is the pathway for the nerves running between the brain and the body, and is easily injured.

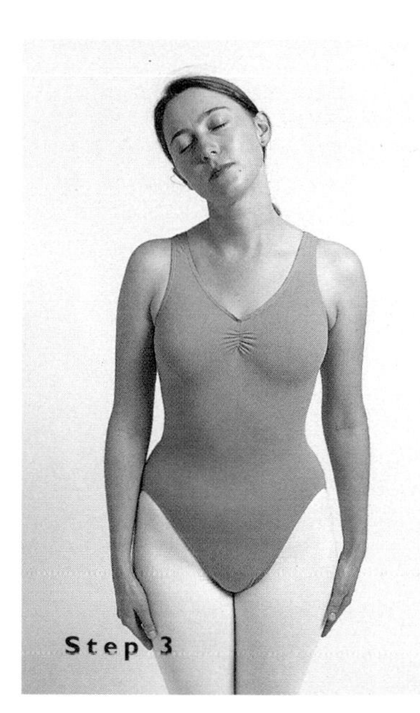
Step 3

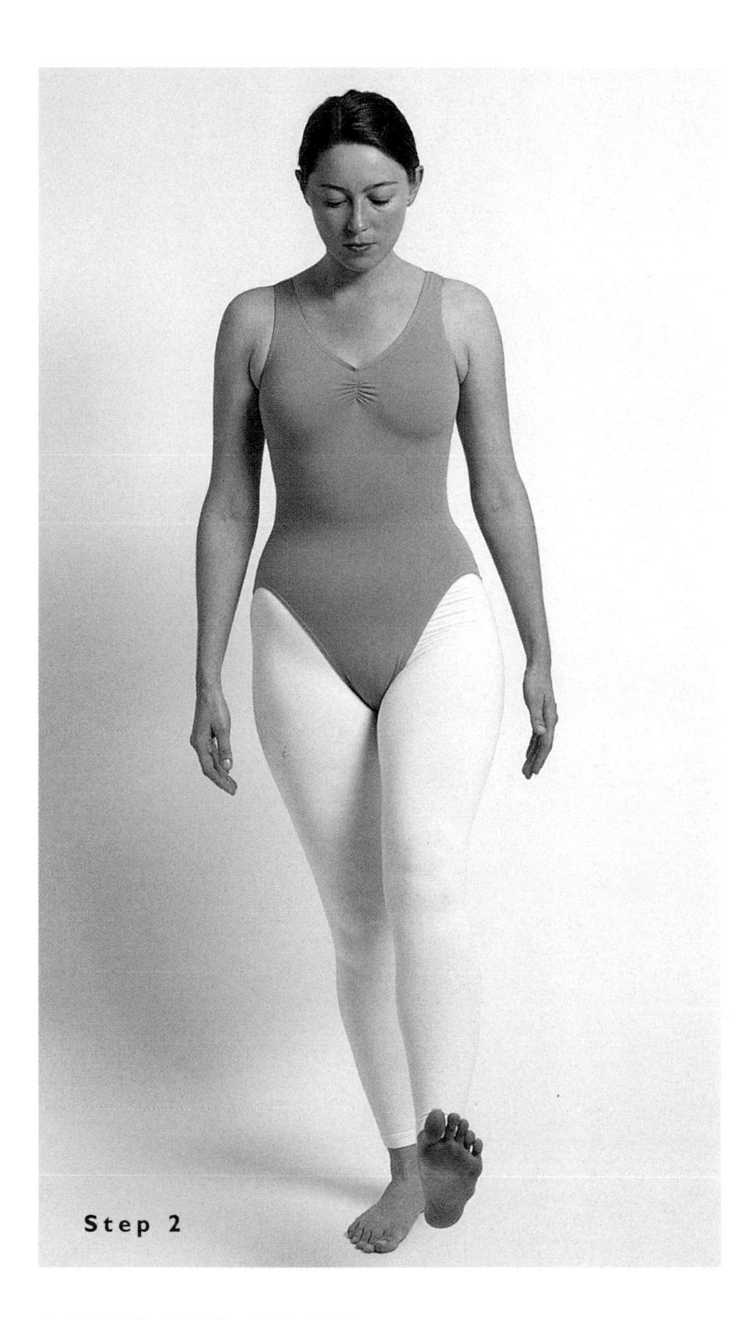
Step 2

ANKLE AND WRIST ROTATIONS

1. Stand with your body balanced. Raise your arms in front of you until they are level with the shoulders. Slowly rotate the wrists in a clockwise direction, then anticlockwise. Feel the energy moving through your arms.

2. Return your arms to your side. Balance on one leg while extending the other in front. The foot need not be lifted far from the floor. Circle the ankle in both directions.

3. Repeat with the other leg. You may prefer to do these exercises sitting on the floor with your legs stretched in front of you.

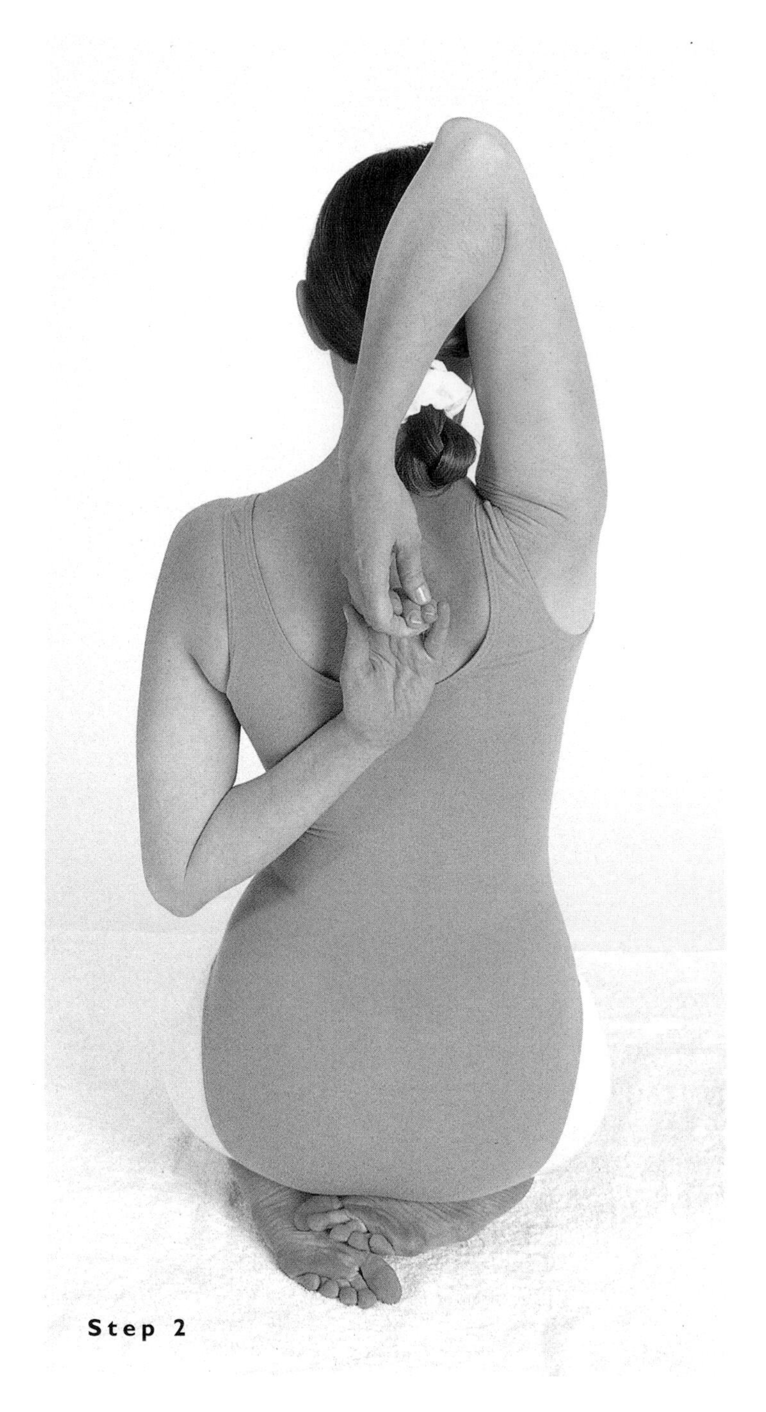

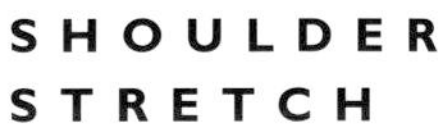

Step 2

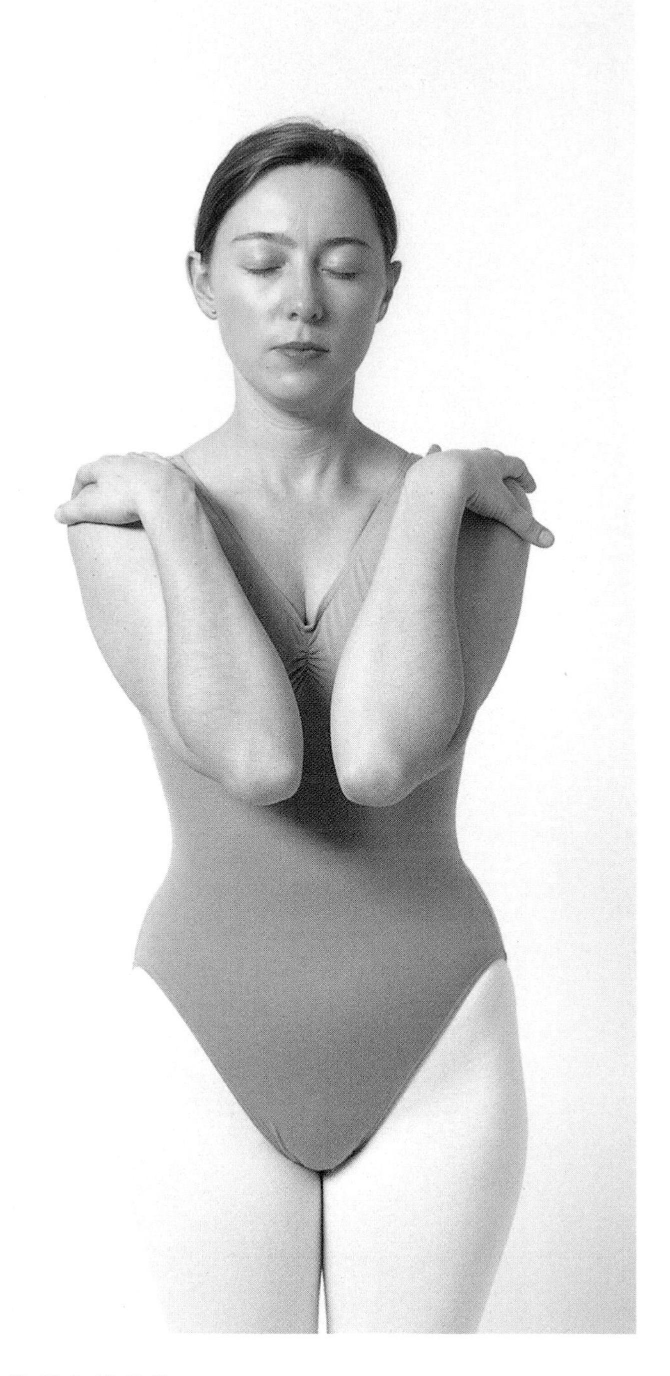

SHOULDER STRETCH

1. In a sitting or standing position, raise your right arm and bend it so the right elbow is near your right ear and your hand is reaching down your back.

2. Now bend your left arm so the left elbow is near your waist and your hand is reaching up your back. If possible, clasp the two hands. You will feel the stretch in the right shoulder blade. Repeat for the other side.

SHOULDER ROTATION

To lubricate and release tension from tired shoulder joints, rotations are excellent.

1. Place your hands on your shoulders and make large, slow circles with your elbows in a clockwise direction.

2. Repeat in an anticlockwise direction.

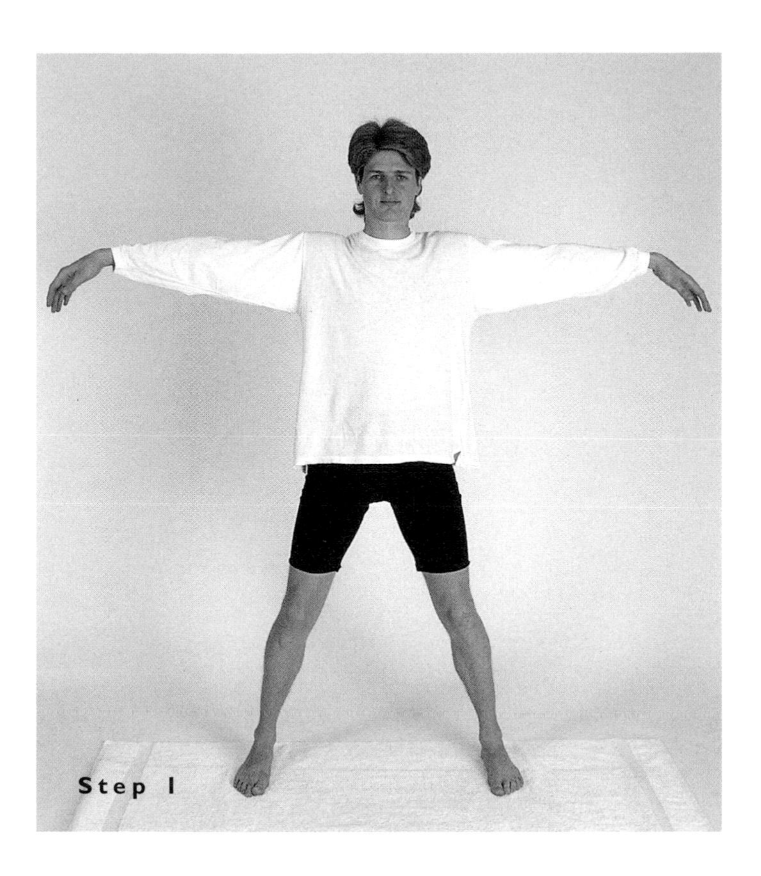

FLOPPY TWIST

This twist loosens the whole body. Allow the knees to bend with the movement and keep the elbows soft.

1. Stand with your legs about 3 feet (1 m) apart and your feet parallel. Raise arms outwards at shoulder level and bend the knees slightly.

2. Twist your body to one side in a loose "ragdoll" fashion, so that your hands softly slap your back. Now twist to the other side.

3. Keep twisting from side to side, creating a smooth flowing motion.

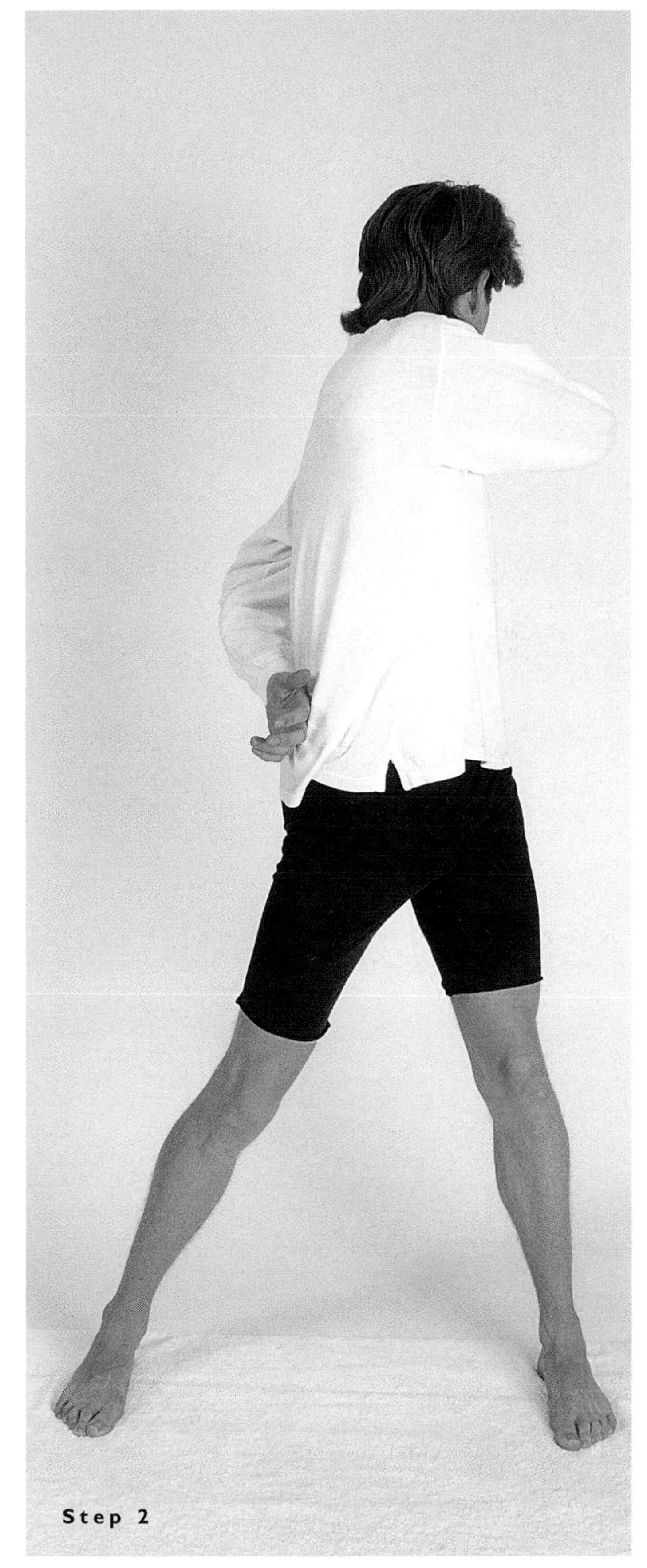

Standing postures

MOUNTAIN

TADASANA

REST

The Mountain pose is the classic resting position for the standing postures. Return to the Mountain to regain balance and stillness between postures.

1. Stand with your feet 3 or 4 inches (9–11 cms) apart. Keep the weight evenly balanced on each foot. Now move the weight slightly towards the outside of each foot, so the arches are raised.

2. Let your arms fall loosely at your sides and look straight ahead.Your head should be aligned with the spine, shoulders held back.

3. Now relax into the position and be steady, still and tall — like a mountain. Do not tighten the face muscles.

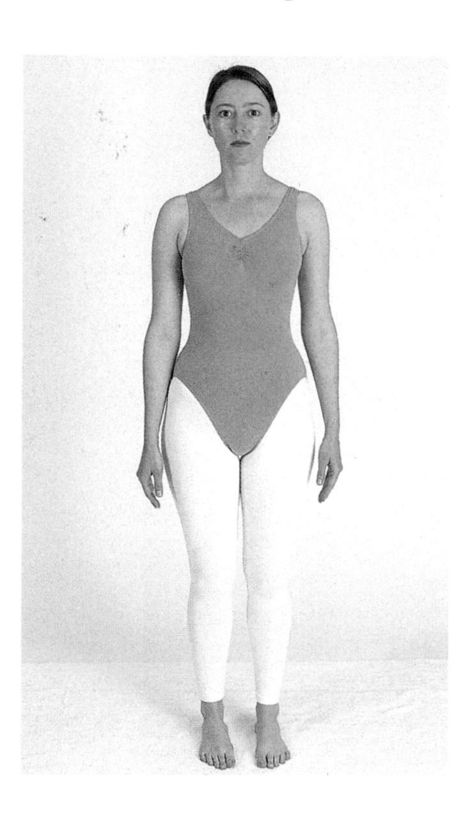

Resting between postures brings continuity to the practice of yoga. A quiet moment of reflection, connecting one posture to the next.

Variation

For an extra stretch, try raising your arms above your head with the fingers linked and palms facing upwards.

Lengthen your whole body and if you can, lift your heels off the floor.

Awareness

Imagine there is a string running through your spine, your body evenly balanced each side of the string. If you were cut in half, both sides would be identical.

Lengthen the spine and neck upwards — this is a subtle movement but you will be able to perceive the sense of space it creates. You will suddenly feel much taller.

Benefits

- creates harmony in the body
- aligns the body
- improves posture
- encourages physical "awareness"
- stills the mind

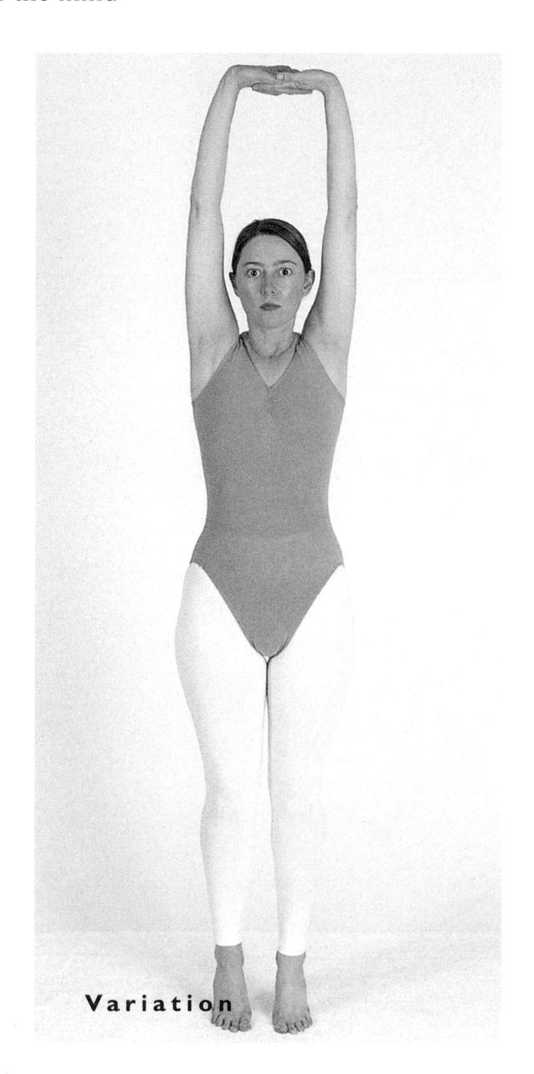

Variation

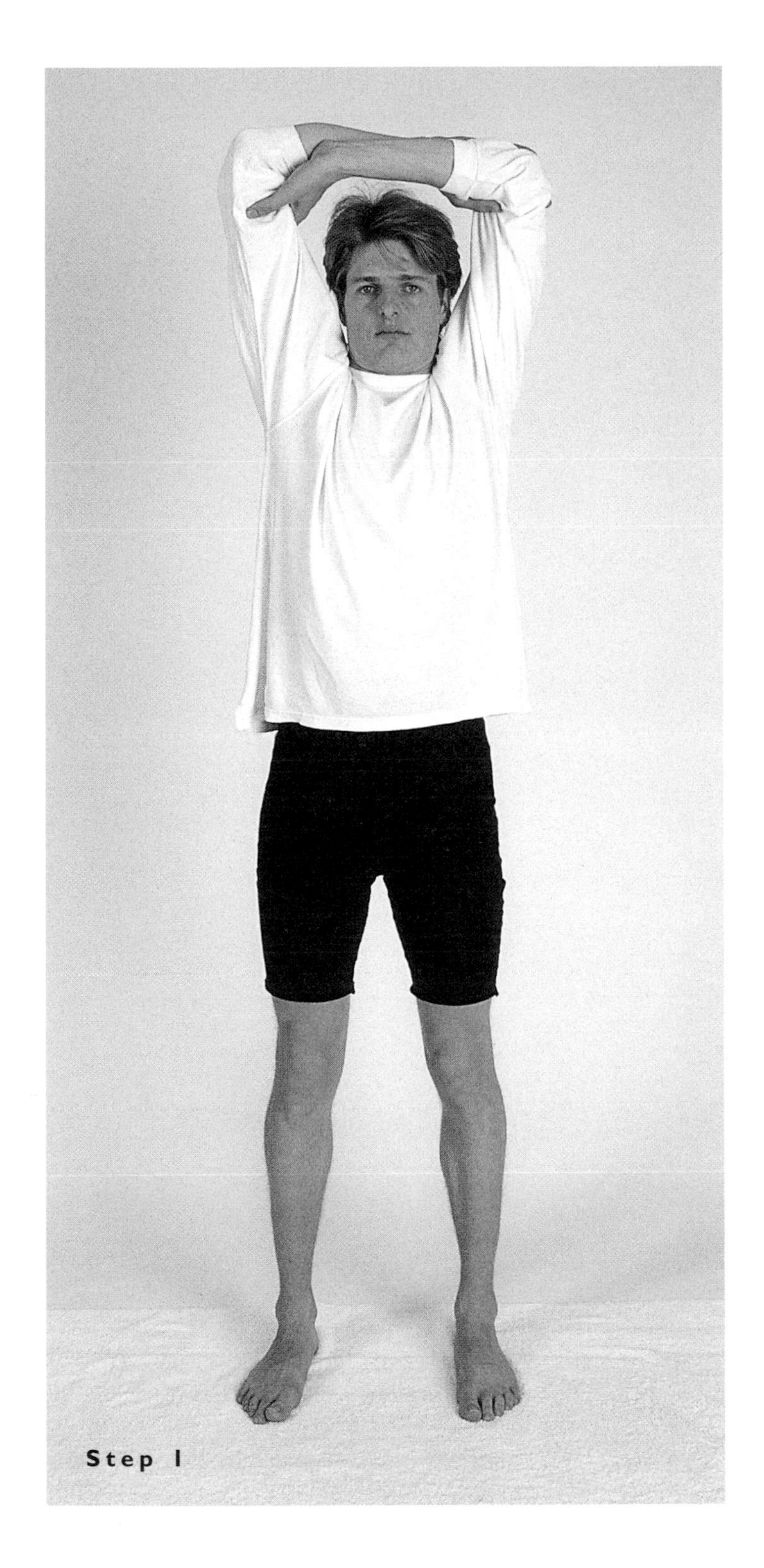

FORWARD BEND

UTTANASANA

REST

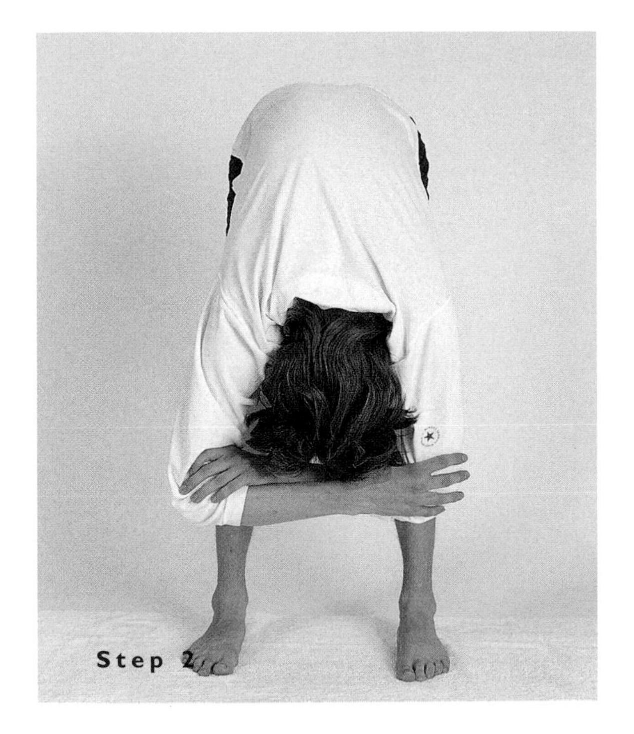

Uttanasana is an alternative resting pose in which the body hangs forward. It is wonderfully relaxing and works gently to elongate the spine and neck. It is also very rejuvenating as it reverses the normal body position — the top half hangs down, while the bottom half extends up.

1. Stand with the feet about hip width apart. Inhale, raise your arms and fold until each hand is clasping the elbow of the other arm. Stretch your upper torso towards the ceiling.
2. Exhale and, moving from the hips, let your upper torso hang downwards. Relax your head and neck, but keep your legs stretched upwards so your buttocks are reaching towards the ceiling. Remain in the position and continue breathing steadily.

Awareness

Remember to hold the knees straight. Check your legs are not sloping backwards — keeping the weight towards the front of the feet will help. Enjoy the sensation of not having to support your upper torso. Let the back muscles totally relax.

Benefits

- relaxes the back muscles
- stimulates the spinal nerves
- aids indigestion and constipation
- stimulates blood flow to the brain

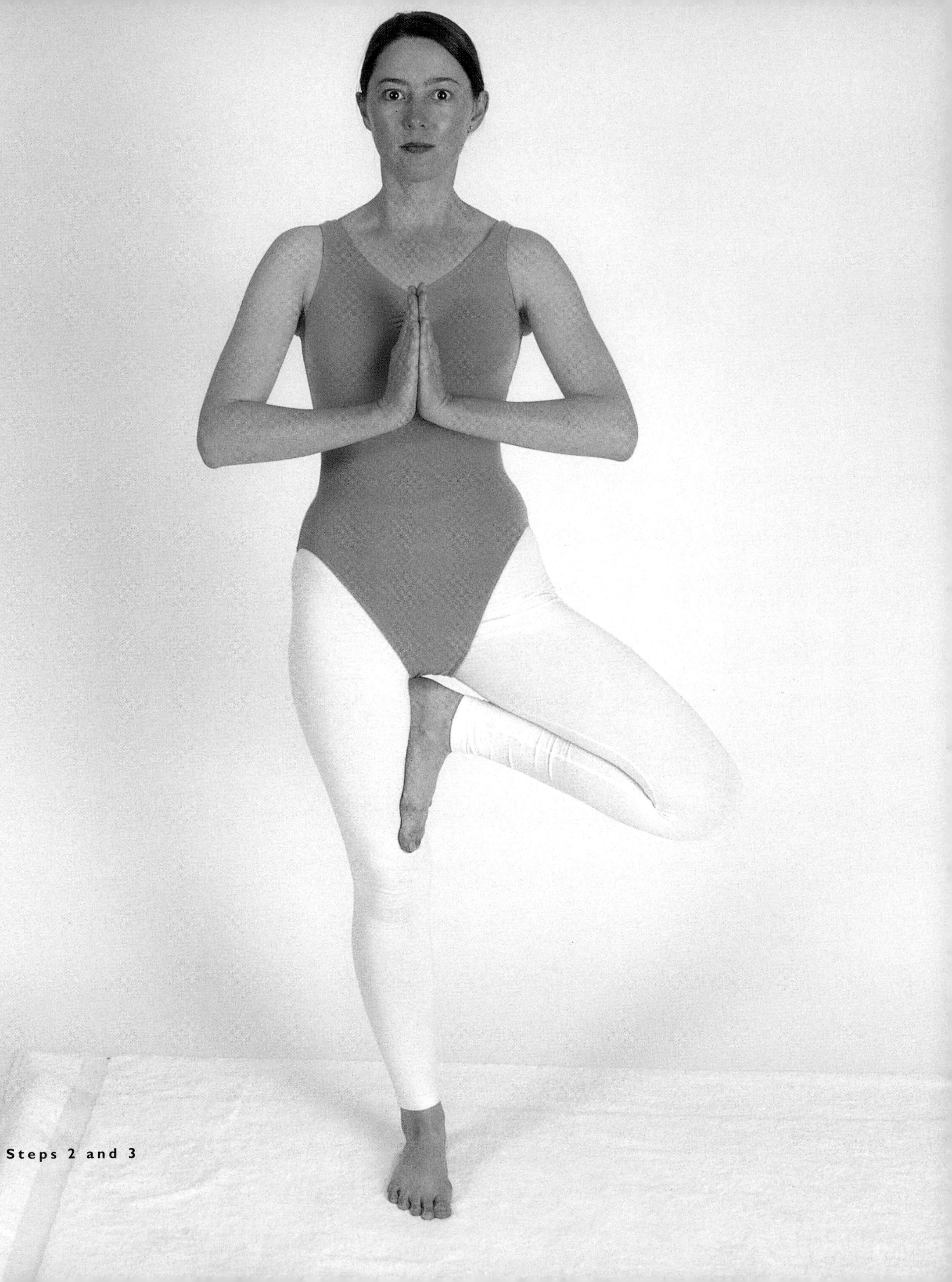

Steps 2 and 3

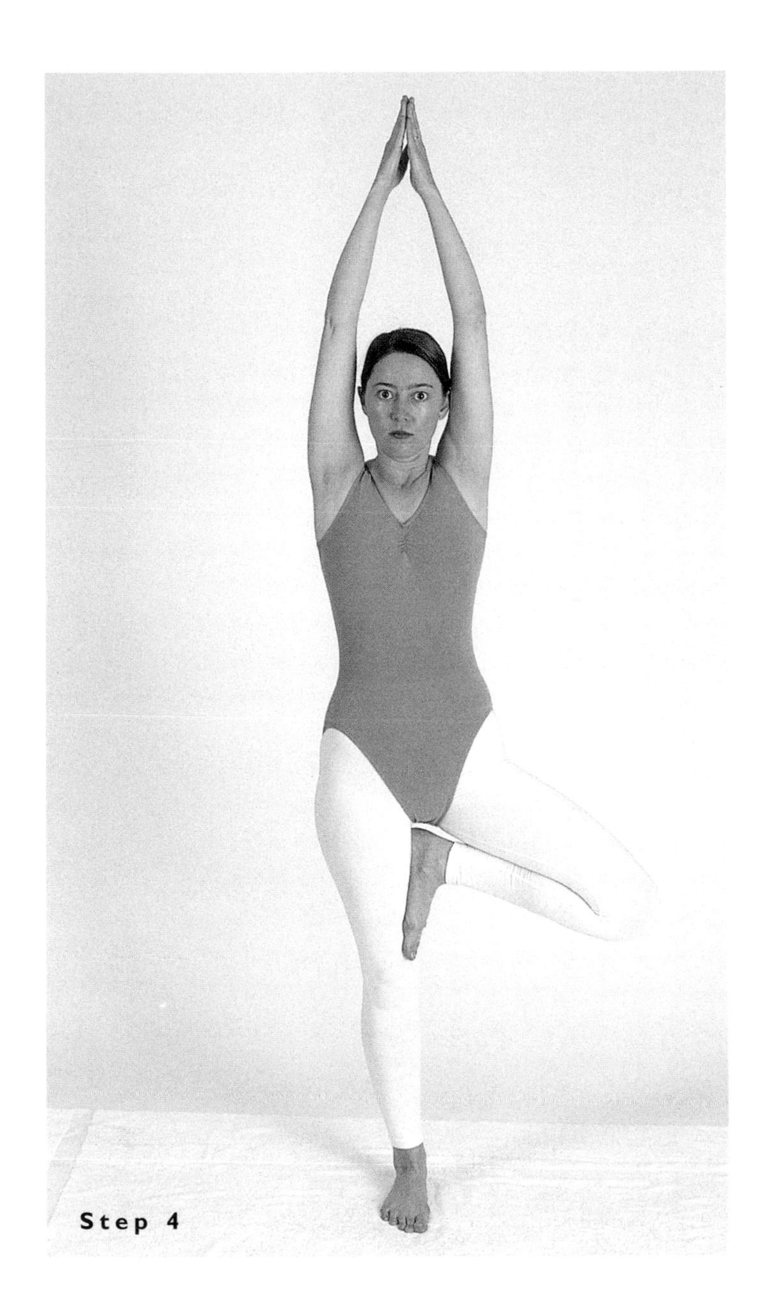
Step 4

Balance poses develop co-ordination,
grace and harmony.
The stillness of these postures brings peace
and repose from daily cares.

TREE

VRKSASANA

BALANCE

Balance postures are often very difficult for the beginner. They look simple, but the harmony of mind and body required for these poses comes only with perseverance. However, once you begin, progress is usually swift. Remember, concentration is the key.

Practice on both sides — you may find one side easier than the other. If you are having difficulty, try focusing on a spot very close to you, or stand in front of a mirror. Keep the foot on the floor steady and try not to let the foot or knee roll inwards.

1. Stand with your feet together and hands at your side, as in the Mountain posture (see page 24). Fix your gaze on a spot on the wall in front of you. Keep looking at the spot throughout the whole posture.

2. Bend and raise one leg, so the sole of the foot is resting on the opposite thigh. It is easier if you use your hands to guide the foot into position.

3. Now bring your hands into a prayer position. Keep the breath even and slow. Try to achieve equilibrium, maintaining your gaze at the spot in front of you. If you lose your balance, don't panic — just begin again.

4. Once you can balance in the prayer position, try raising your arms above your head, palms touching. Stretch towards the sky.

Variation

Instead of raising one foot onto the thigh, try placing it directly in front of the other foot — heel to toe.

Benefits

- calms the mind and soothes the nerves
- improves co-ordination and balance
- strengthens the legs and feet
- lengthens the spinal column

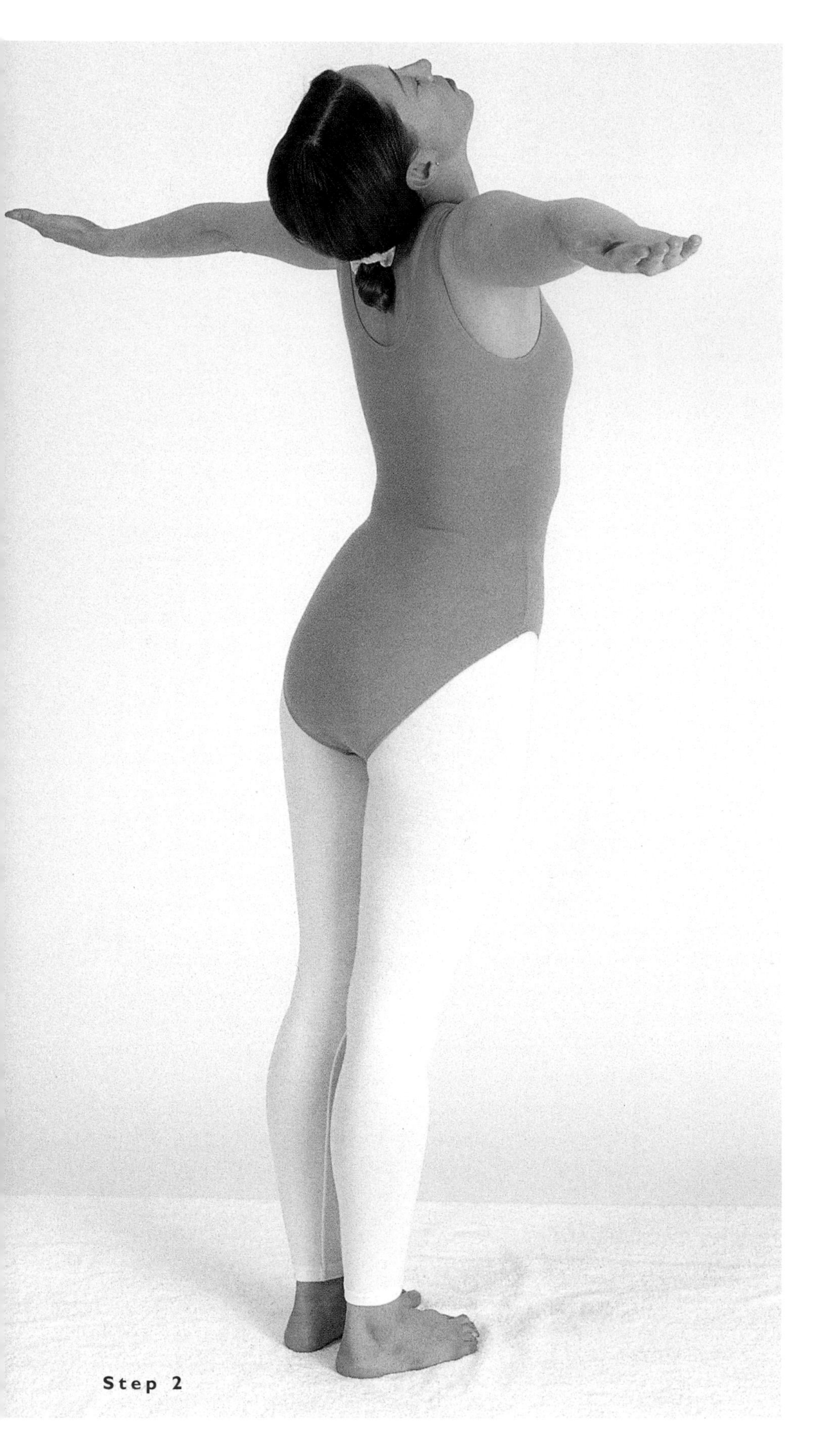

Step 2

PARTING OF THE CLOUDS

BACKWARD BEND

This pose is very soothing and gives a gentle stretch to the rib cage area.

1. Stand in the Mountain posture (see page 24). Inhale, and slowly raise your arms in front of you. Keep the movement loose and soft. Continue to raise your arms until they are above your head, the upper arms in line with your ears.

2. Arch your back and lower your arms to shoulder height, palms facing up. Your neck is reaching towards the ceiling. Imagine the warmth of the sun on your face. Breathe normally. *Do not hold the position for long as you may strain your back.*

3. Exhaling, carefully raise your head to normal position and bring the arms back above your head.

4. Conclude by gently lowering your arms in front of your body.

5. Repeat the posture, concentrating on creating one slow, smooth movement.

Benefits

- opens the rib cage
- stimulates digestive organs
- releases energy in the throat area

Caution

If you have high blood pressure, avoid stretching too far backwards. Do not hold the final position. If you feel at all dizzy, do not practice the posture. Consult a teacher.

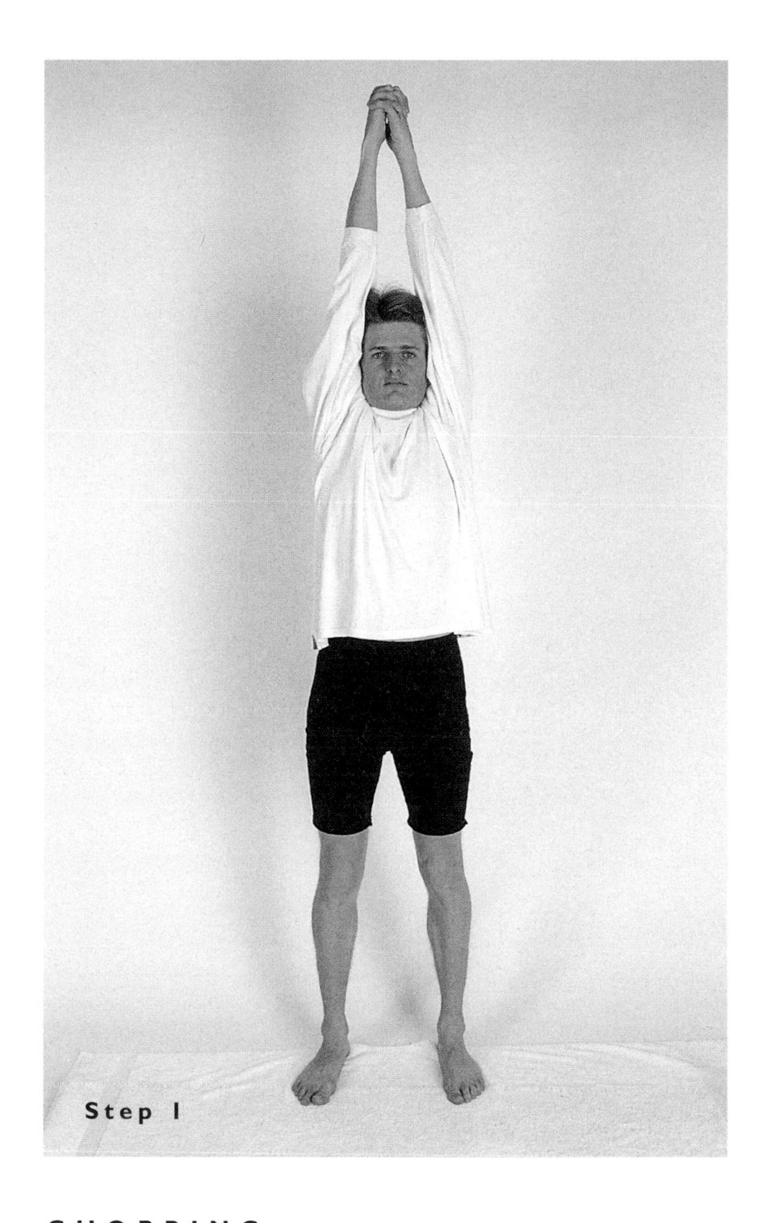

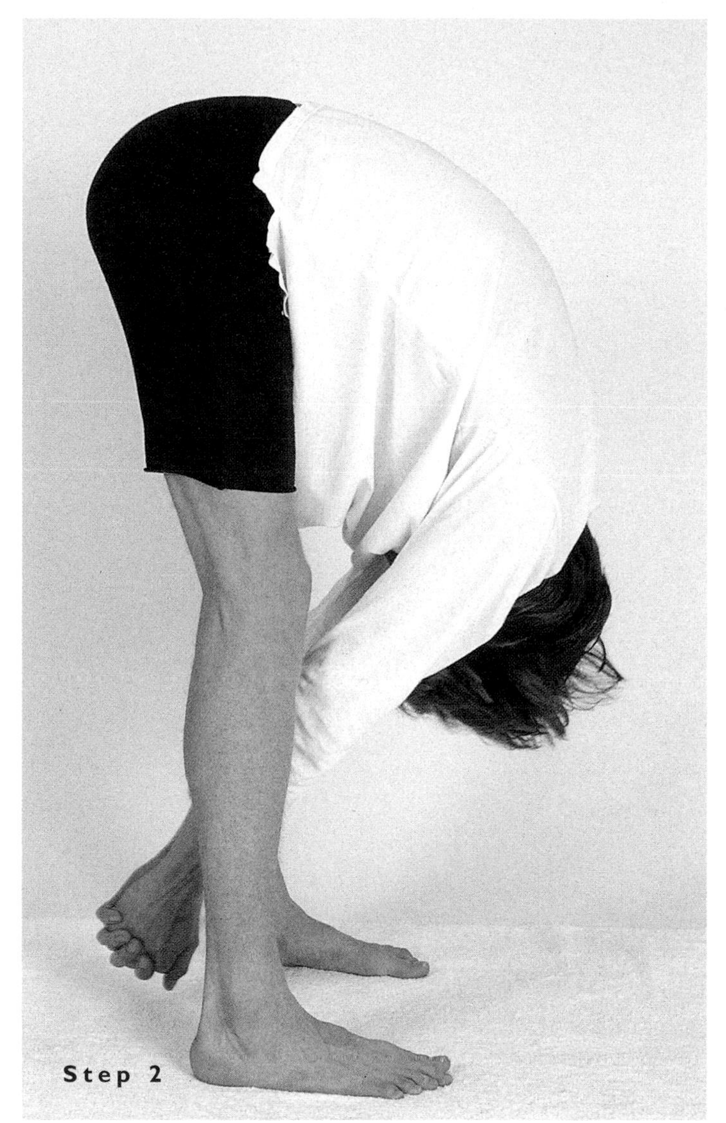

CHOPPING WOOD

LOOSENER/FORWARD BEND

Chopping Wood releases stored tension and awakens energy in the body.

1. Place feet shoulder width apart. Inhale, clasp your hands together and stretch your arms above your head.

2. Now, exhaling strongly in a "puff", drop your upper torso down from the hips so your hands swing between your legs. Keep your arms straight. The downward movement is a single action — do not bounce.

3. Pretend you are chopping with an axe. Raise your arms and torso, then repeat the movement. As you chop downwards, let all tension or negative feelings be expelled from your body.

Benefits

- releases tension
- stimulates energy flow
- tones the chest muscles

Remember to practice forward bends after backward bends. The forward posture helps the back muscles unwind and lengthen.

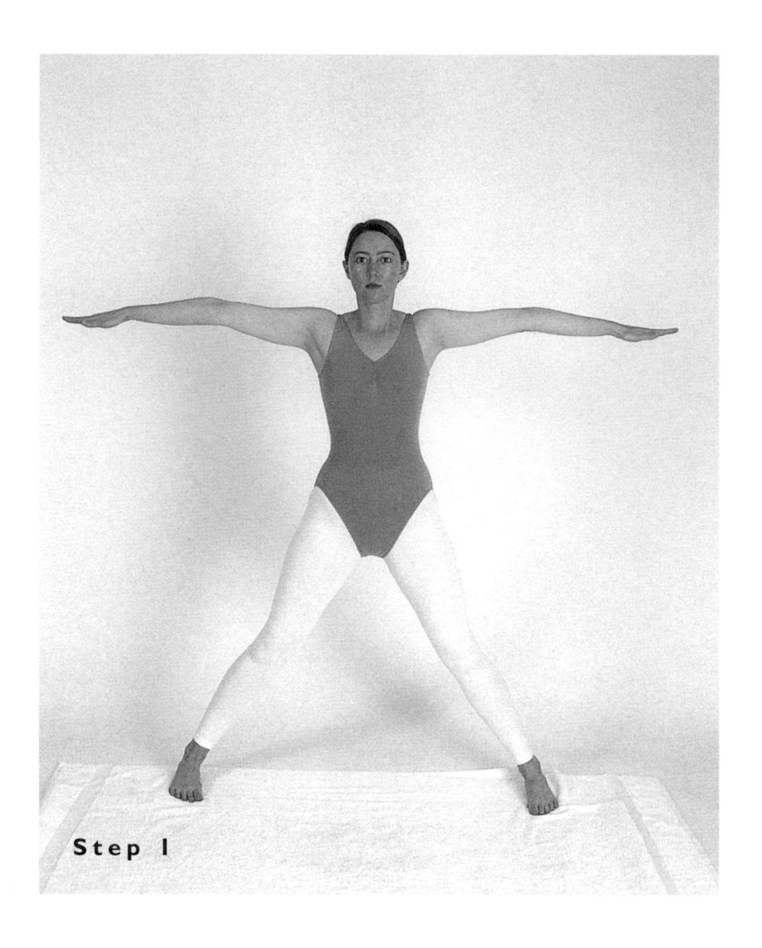
Step 1

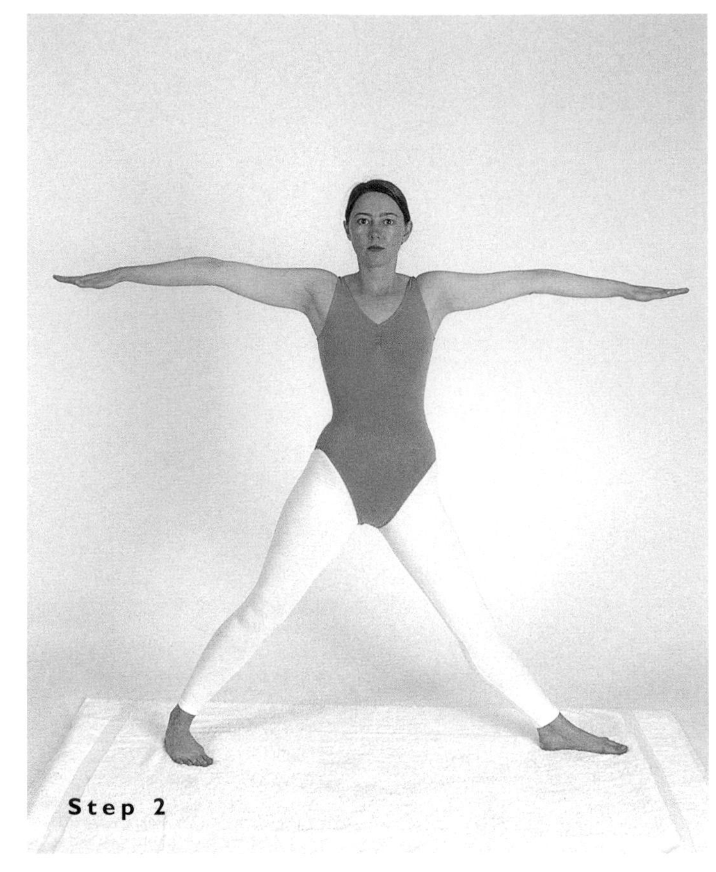
Step 2

TRIANGLE

TRIKONASANA

STRETCH

The sideways stretch of the Triangle pose helps to align the spine and promotes a strong body. You will feel an increase in vitality after this practice.

1. Stand with feet wide apart — about 3 to 4 feet (1 m) — toes pointing forward. Take the time to check your whole body is aligned; your feet should be parallel and hips straight. Raise your arms outward at shoulder height and stretch from chest to fingertips. Make sure your arms form one line. Look straight ahead.

2. Reposition your feet so that the right foot is turned inwards slightly and the left is facing the side wall. In this position, the whole left leg is now facing the side wall. The heel of the left foot should be in line with the arch of the right. Ensure you feel steady and comfortable in the position and then inhale.

3. As you exhale, bend from the hips, not the waist, towards the left side. It is important to try and remain in a straight line — do not lean forwards. Lower your left hand onto the shin, ankle or floor, whichever is comfortable, keeping your arm straight.

4. Raise your right arm until it is in line with your left arm. Rotate your trunk until it faces forwards by swivelling your right hip backwards.

5. Look up at the right fingertips, keeping your head aligned with the spine. If this is uncomfortable, look straight ahead. The arms, left leg and torso now form the three sides of a triangle. Breathe normally in the posture for a few seconds, then carefully return to the upright position. Bending the knees as you come out of the posture prevents back strain.

6. Repeat for other side. After completing the Triangle, rest in Forward Bend posture (see page 25).

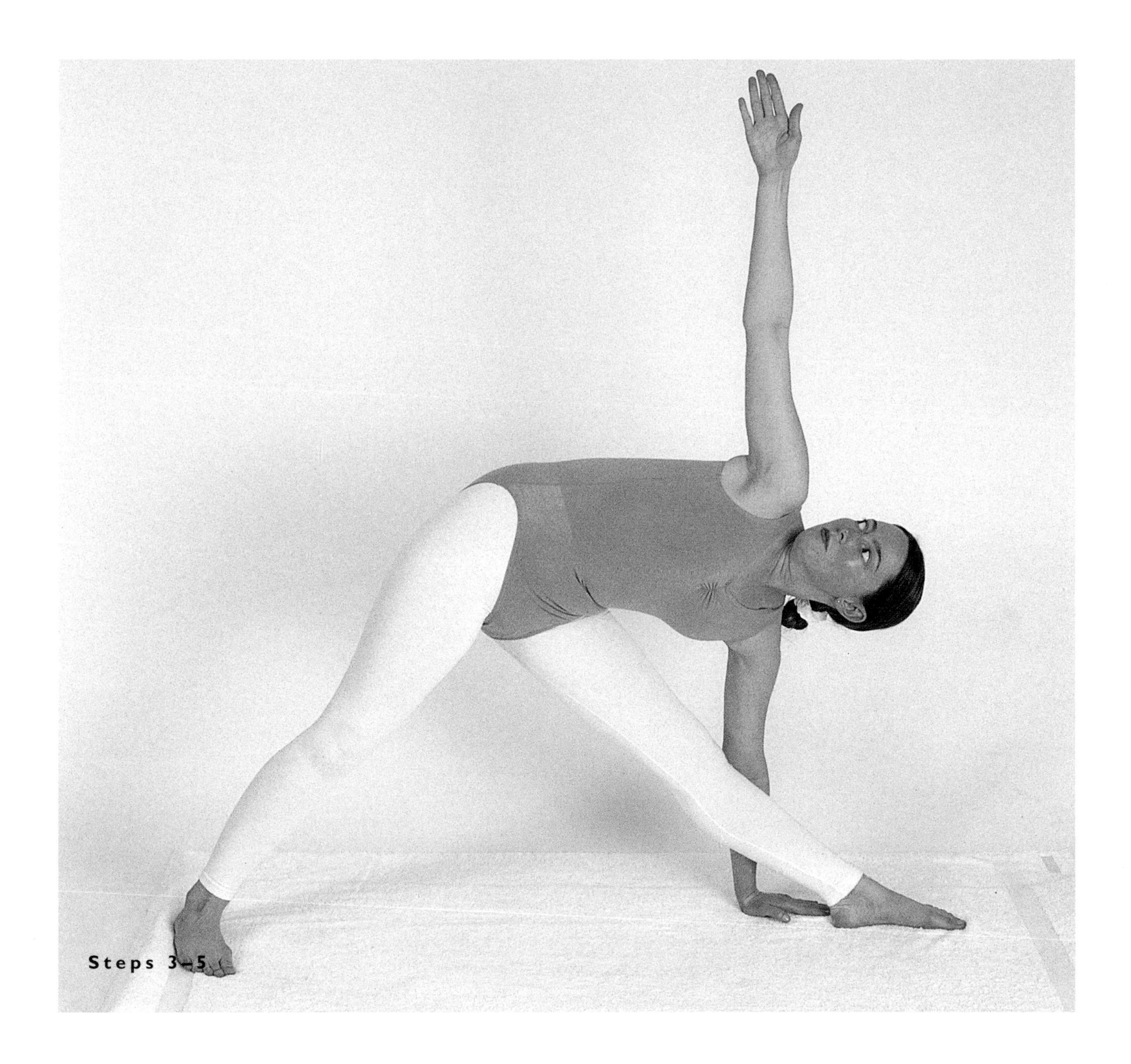
Steps 3–5

Variation
If you are finding this posture difficult, try bending the leg facing the wall. This should ease some strain.

Do not try to force your hand too far down the leg when you first try this practice. Practicing the posture against a wall will help keep your body aligned.

Benefits
- increases vital energy
- stimulates the nervous system
- aligns the spine
- strengthens the muscles
- improves flexibility

Caution
This posture is very strong — be careful not to strain your body in any way. If you are experiencing pain or discomfort, come out of the posture and rest.

Avoid this practice if you have high blood pressure, heart problems, are menstruating or during pregnancy.

TWISTING TRIANGLE

PARIVRTTA TRIKONASANA

TWIST

This posture greatly enhances the flexibility of the hips. It is very refreshing, especially if performed dynamically. Repeat the whole process several times, either slowly or dynamically. *Lengthen the spine and pivot at the hips*. Such subtle concepts are intrinsic to yoga practice, and help you to move much more freely.

1. Stand with feet about 3 feet (1 m) apart, arms at shoulder height, as in Mountain posture, position 1 (see page 24).

2. Bending from the hips, lower your upper torso until it forms a right angle with your legs. Gaze straight ahead.

3. Swivel your torso, touching your left foot with your right hand. Your left arm should be straight. Look up at your left hand.

4. Now, twist to the other side to touch your right foot with your left hand.

5. Return to position 2, where your body forms a right angle with your legs.

6. Raise your body back into position 1. Repeat the whole process.

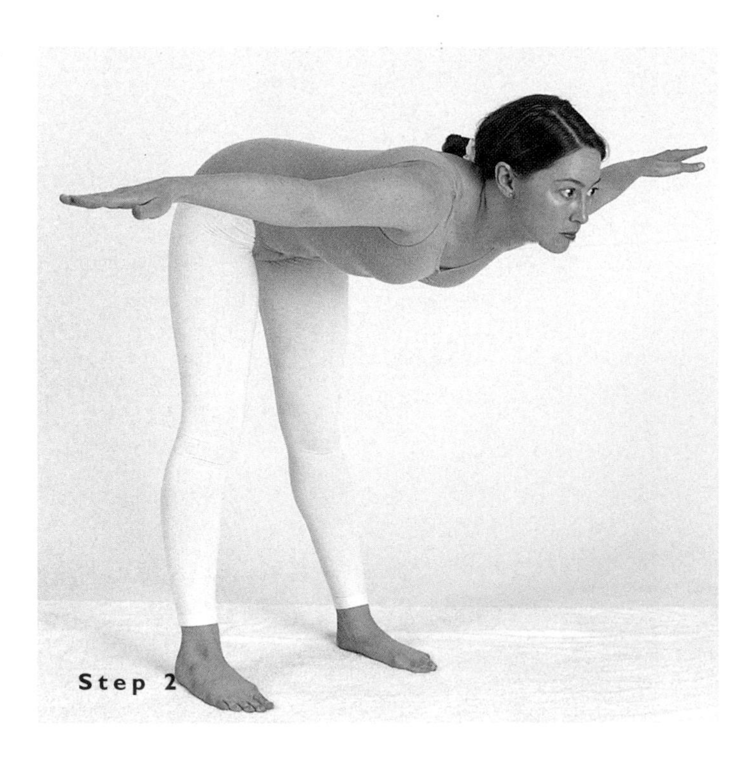

Step 2

Awareness

In position 2, where your body is stretched forward, concentrate on lengthening and straightening the spine. You can do this by pushing your buttocks back and stretching forward from the base of the spine. Imagine a space forming between each of the vertebrae, beginning at the base of the spine. Notice how you can pivot at the hips.

You will probably feel a tightening of the hamstring muscles in the backs of your knees. Enjoy developing a new sense of flexibility.

Benefits

- stimulates the nervous system
- aids digestion
- tones abdominal organs
- relieves constipation
- increases flexibility
- strengthens back muscles
- helps relieve depression and anxiety

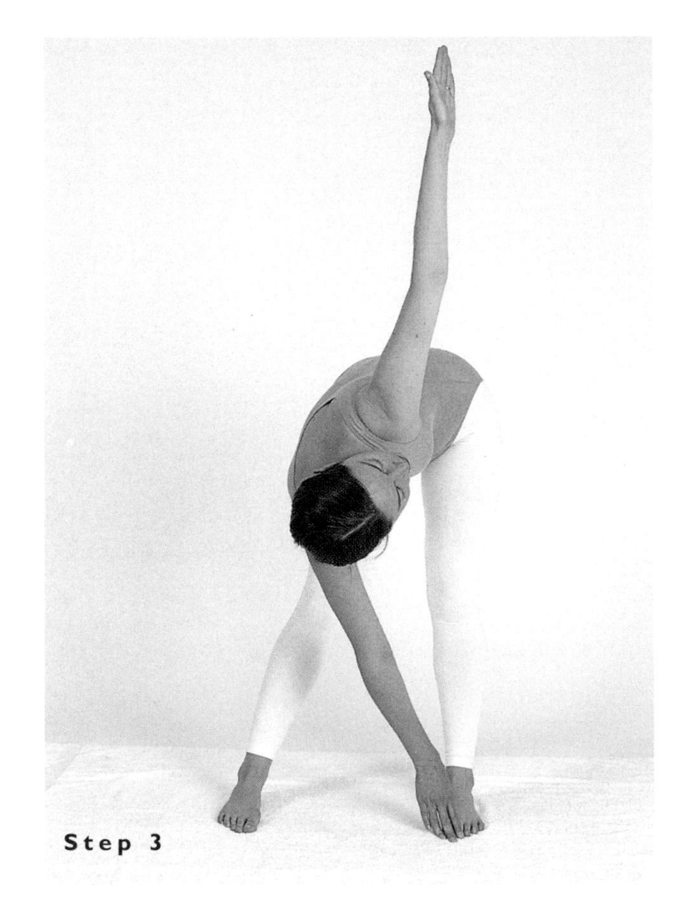

Step 3

Sitting postures

THUNDERBOLT

VAJRASANA

REST

Many sitting and floor postures begin and end in the Thunderbolt or the Hero pose. Choose the posture your body prefers. Rest in either pose to soothe the legs.

1. Sit on your heels with the knees held close together.

2. Cross the toes of one foot with the other, so one foot rests in the other. The toes are touching and the heels are apart. Rest your hands on your thighs or in your lap, whichever is comfortable. Lengthen the spine and hold your head upright, looking straight ahead. This is known as the Thunderbolt pose.

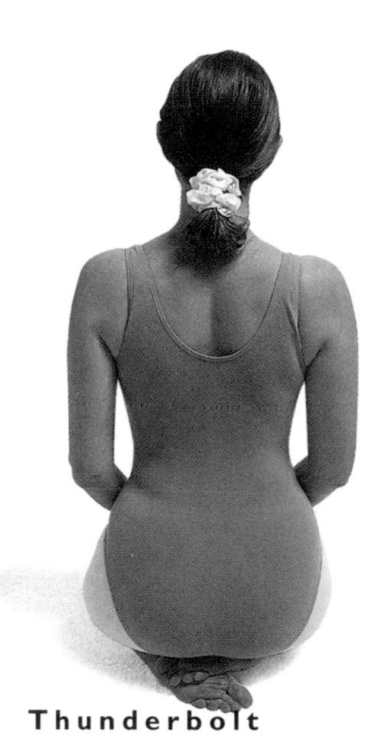

Thunderbolt

Benefits

- gently stretches knee joints, ankle joints and inner thighs
- improves the functioning of the digestive system
- aids indigestion
- strengthens pelvic muscles
- encourages deep breathing by opening the chest area
- calms the mind

Caution

Take care in these positions if you have weak or injured knees. Do not force the postures or remain in them for too long. A folded blanket under the knees may help.

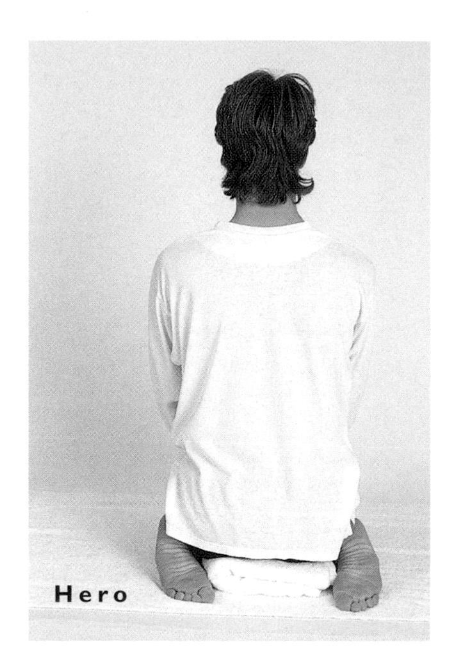

Hero

HERO

VIRASANA

REST

1.Sitting in the Thunderbolt position, separate the feet so your buttocks lower towards the floor. If you find your buttocks cannot reach the floor, place a folded towel or blanket beneath them to prevent you from straining.

2. Position the feet so they are in a straight line, resting near your hips. Try to keep the knees together. This is the Hero pose.

Variation

This posture is known as Supta Virasana. From the Hero pose, you can stretch the whole body by leaning back on the floor. First lower yourself onto the elbows and then carefully lower your back and head to the floor. Try to keep the knees together — this may be difficult at first. Stretch your arms above your head. Breathe steadily. To get up again, raise your body back onto the elbows.

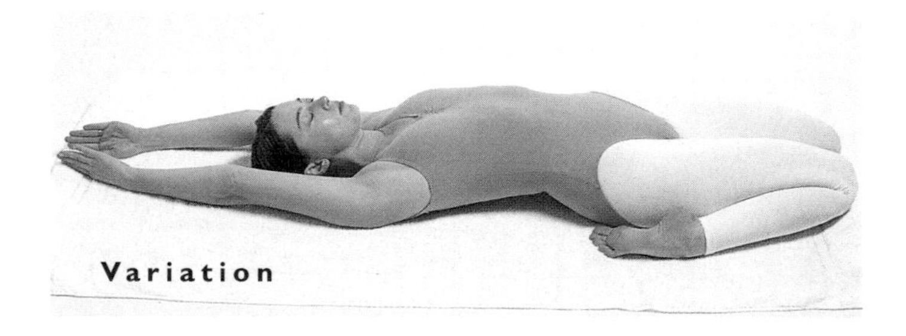

Variation

CHILD

PINDASANA

REST

The Child pose is another resting position. Notice how all the muscles unwind in this posture. Particularly soothing for tight back muscles and after backbending postures.

1. Sit in the Thunderbolt pose (see page 33). Inhale.
2. Exhale, gently bend forward until your head is resting on the floor. Breathe steadily. Let your back arch naturally and comfortably. Rest your arms on the floor with your palms facing upwards.

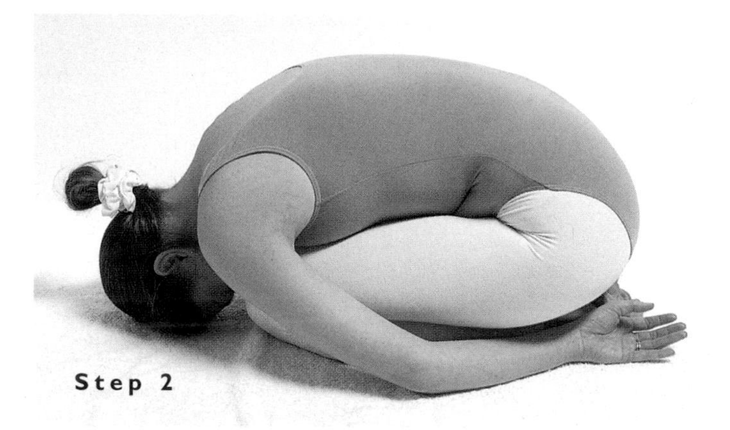

Step 2

Variation
Stretch your arms out in front of you, palms facing downwards. Feel the extension of the back muscles.

Awareness
As you rest in the Child pose, observe how the posture affects you. The body, the mind and the soul are nourished. If you are experiencing anxiety or feeling depleted in any way, try taking "time out" in the Child. The posture is that of the baby in the womb.

Benefits
- calms the mind and emotions
- restores energy
- stretches and soothes back muscles
- tones the pelvic region and sexual organs
- regulates adrenal gland function
- soothes sciatica

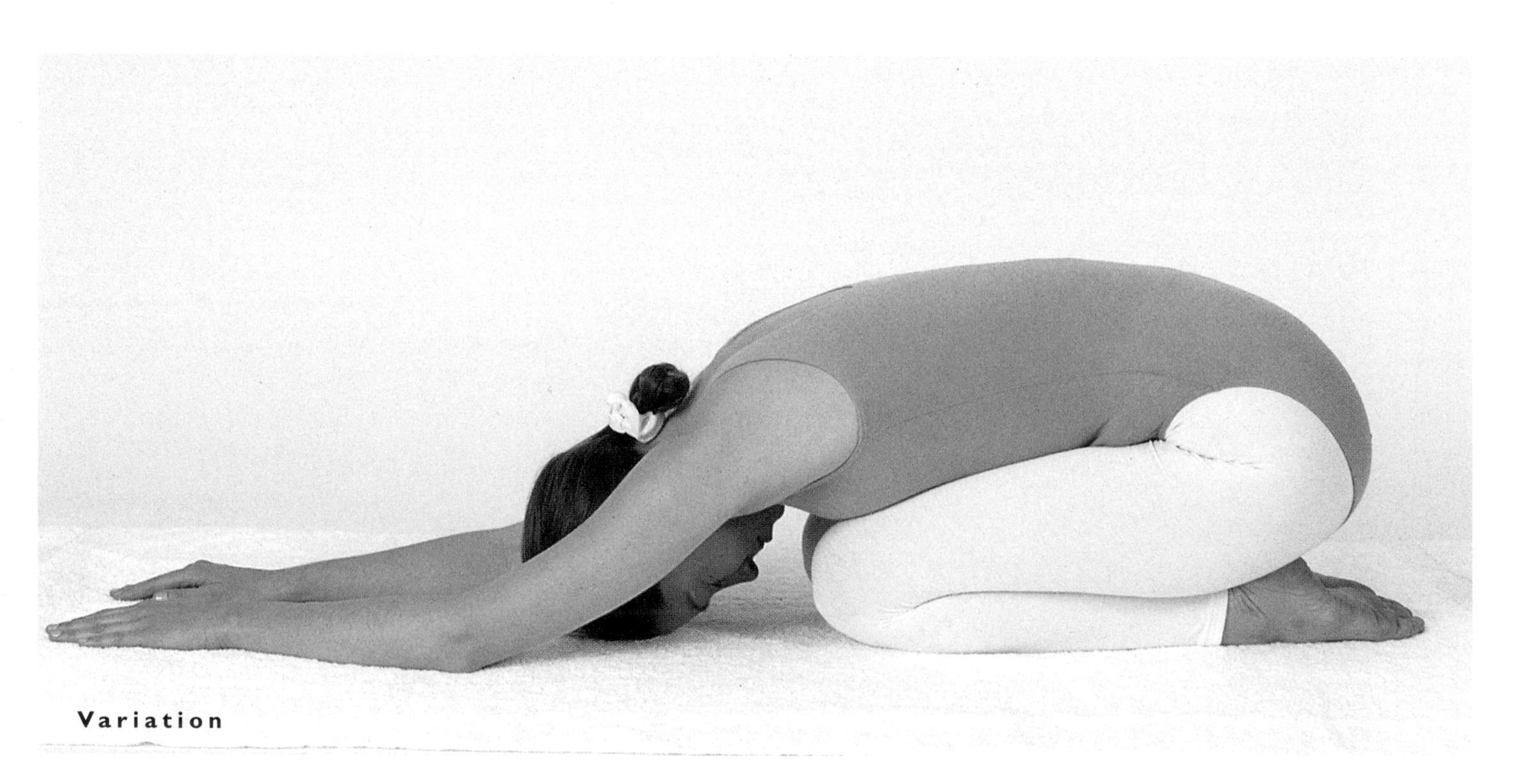

Variation

BUTTERFLY

BADDHA KONASANA

LOOSENER

Loosening postures lubricate stiff joints and ease tight muscles. You will feel a fresh surge of energy awaken in your body.

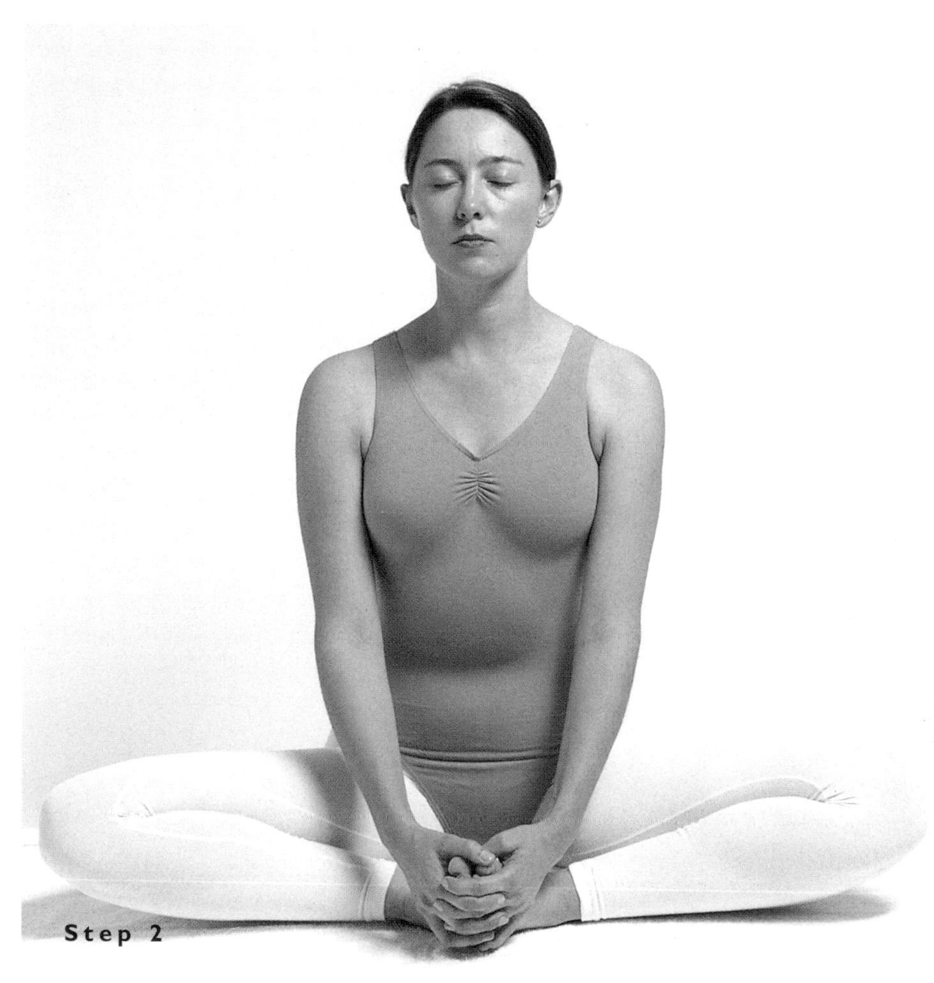

Step 2

In the Western world, we are often very stiff in the hip joints. Work gently to free the joints and enjoy an increase in mobility and flexibility. The Butterfly posture is an excellent loosening exercise. A cushion or folded blanket under the buttocks will help when you are first practicing this posture.

1. Sit on the floor and bend your legs so the feet are joined sole to sole.

2. Grasp the feet and bring them as close to your body as possible as shown.

3. Place your hands on your knees and gently push them towards the floor. Feel your thighs widen.

4. Release the knees, then push them downwards again. Each time you repeat the movement you will feel the joints give way a little more.

5. Once you have some flexibility in the joints, try the movement without the help of your hands. Let the knees move up and down in a smooth motion, like the wings of a butterfly.

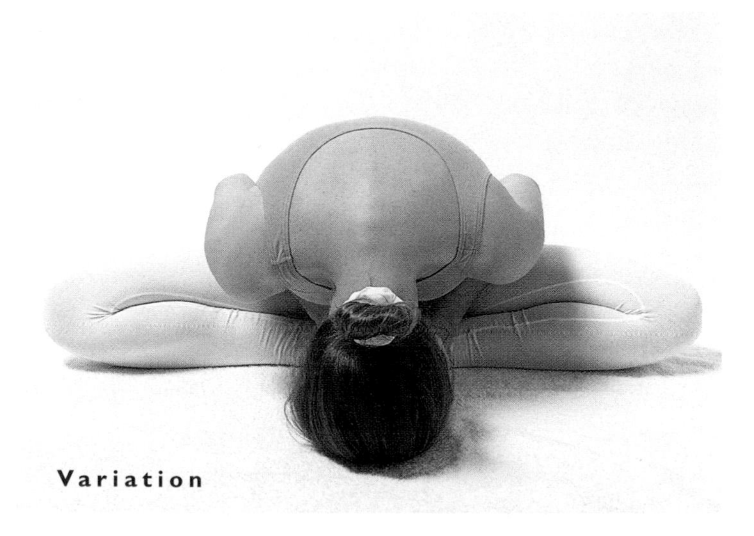

Variation

Variation

Sit still in the Butterfly, knees as close to the floor as comfortable. Inhale, then exhale, gently lowering your head to the floor, arching your back. Breathe normally. Ease into the posture, feeling the base of the spine open with each exhalation.

Benefits

- loosens hip joints and pelvic region
- tones the thighs
- balances digestive functions
- excellent for bladder and kidney problems
- relieves period pain
- prevents varicose veins

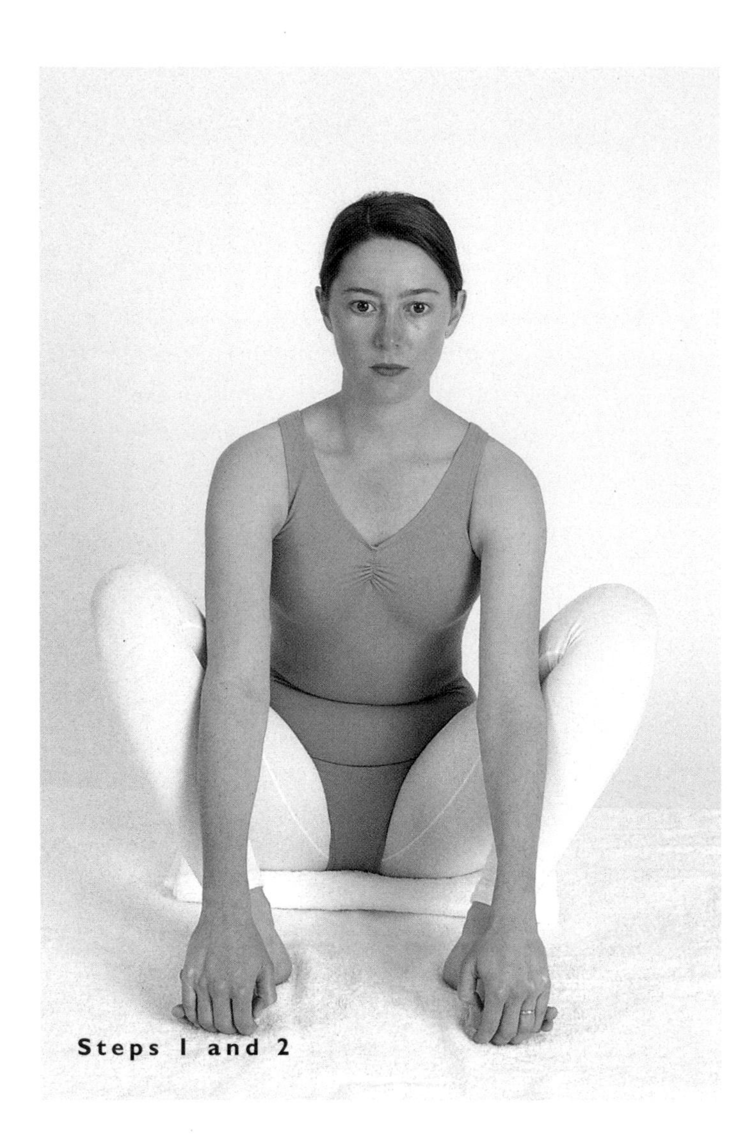
Steps 1 and 2

SEATED BALANCE

MERUDANDASANA

BALANCE

This sitting balance looks daunting, but with a little practice it becomes very easy. Experiment to find the position in which your body is perfectly balanced.

1. Sit with legs bent in front of you, at hip width or a little more. Feet should be flat on the floor. Place a folded towel beneath the buttocks to relieve pressure on the coccyx.
2. Grasp your feet with your hands. Inhale.
3. Holding your breath, raise your legs from the floor, balancing on your buttocks. You will need to lean backwards, but not too far!
4. If you can, straighten your legs and arms. Hold for one or two seconds.
5. Exhale as you lower your legs.

Benefits

- improves balance and concentration
- strengthens the spine and abdominal muscles
- improves posture
- stimulates the internal organs, especially the bladder, reproductive organs and liver
- tones the thighs and firms the buttocks

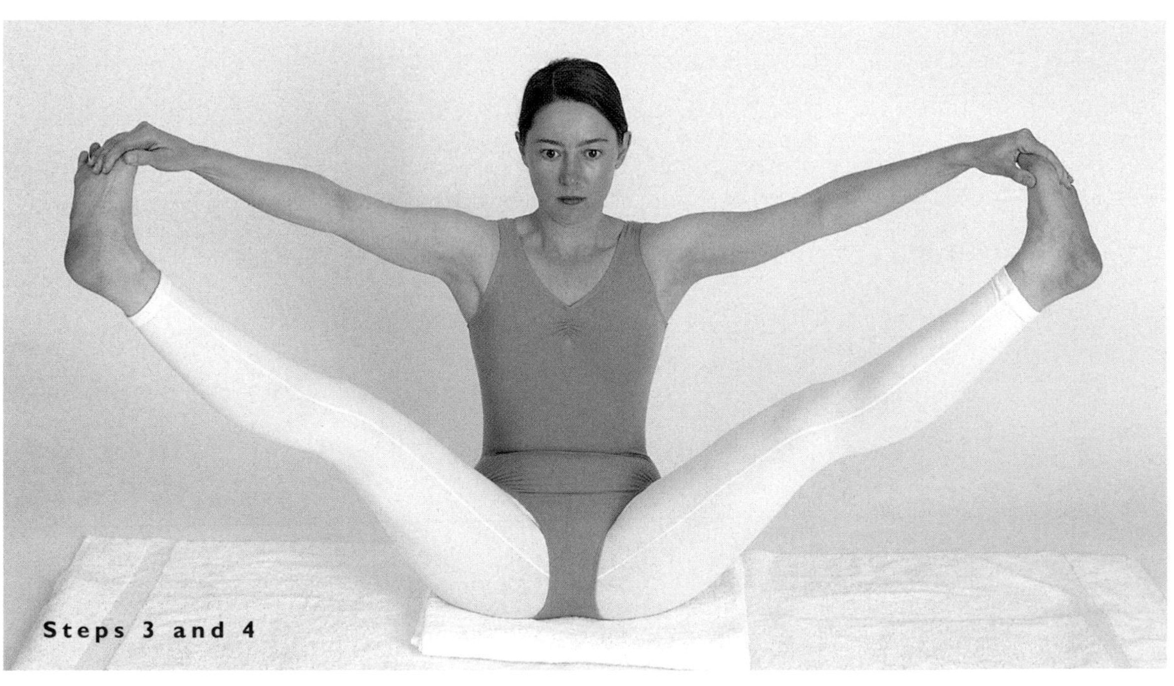
Steps 3 and 4

ARM AND SHOULDER LIFT

YOGA MUDRASANA

STRETCH/FORWARD BEND

Yoga Mudrasana is a classic yoga posture which gently stretches the shoulders and arms, while the body rests.

1. Sit in the Thunderbolt posture (see page 33).
2. Lower your head and place it on the floor in front of your knees. Clasp your hands together, behind your back.
3. Inhale, and begin to lift your arms, hands clasped, away from your back. Push your arms towards your head as far as possible, without strain. Your arms should be in a straight line with your linked hands reaching toward the ceiling. Exhale, then breathe normally in the position for a few moments.
4. Now, inhale again and push your arms even further towards your head. Notice how your body can always stretch a little more than you think possible.
5. Exhale, and lower your arms to rest on the floor. Unwind in the Child pose (see page 34).

Benefits

- stretches the entire shoulder area
- creates space in the spinal column
- rejuvenates the face
- increases energy levels
- activates the immune system

Caution

Work gradually with this posture. Move your arms towards your head as you feel the muscles release. Do not jerk your arms backwards — treat your body with care always.

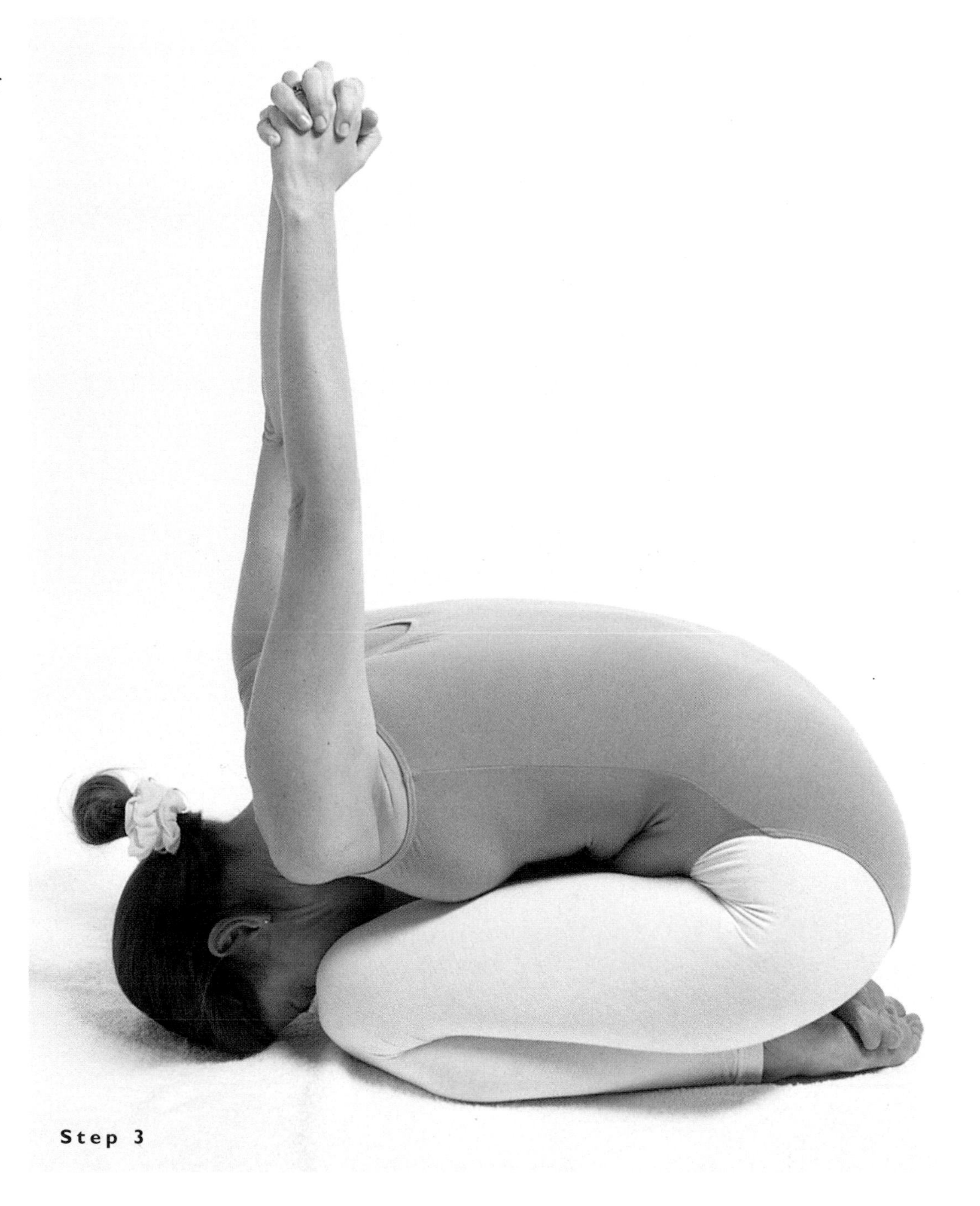

Step 3

HEAD TO KNEE STRETCH

JANU SIRSASANA

STRETCH

Sitting stretches greatly improve flexibility and loosen the pelvic region. Remember to lift and lengthen from the base of the spine. On every exhalation stretch a little more.

You will be surprised at how your tight muscles are willing to unwind.

1. Sit with one leg stretched out in front, the other bent so the foot is resting against your thigh. Try to keep the knee near the floor.

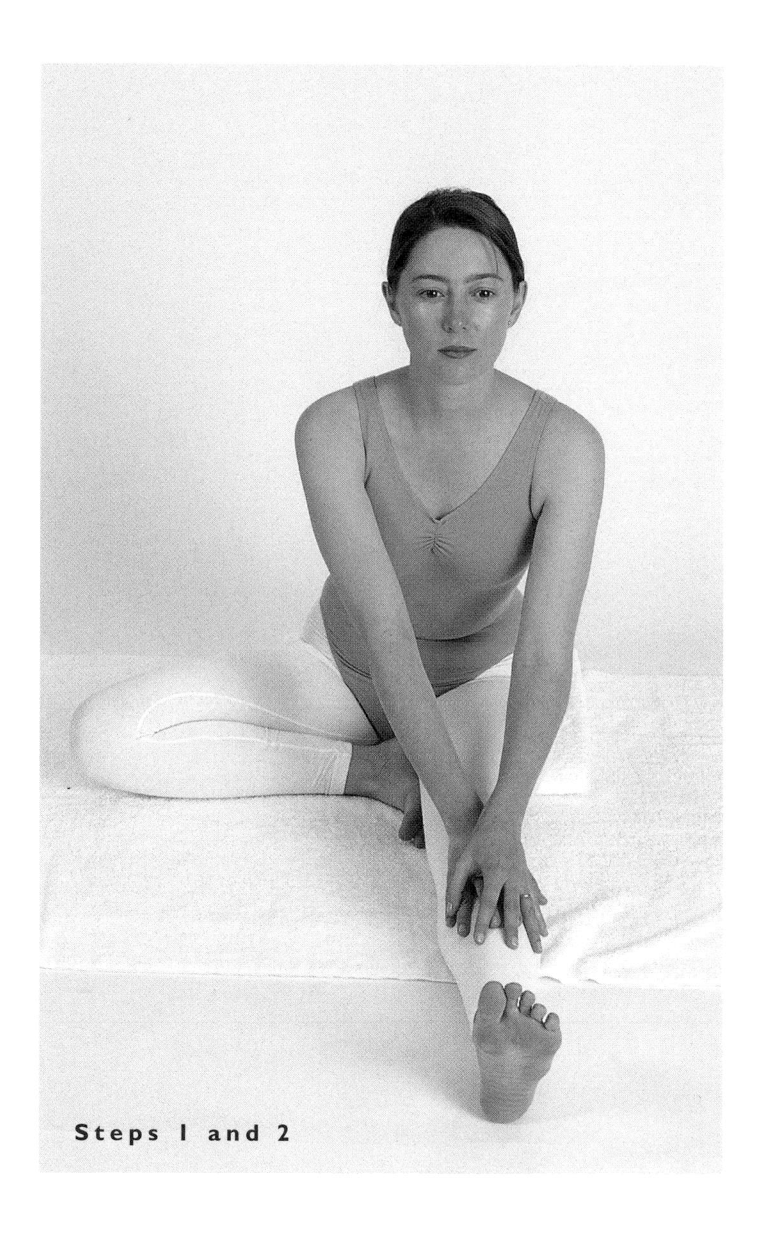

Steps 1 and 2

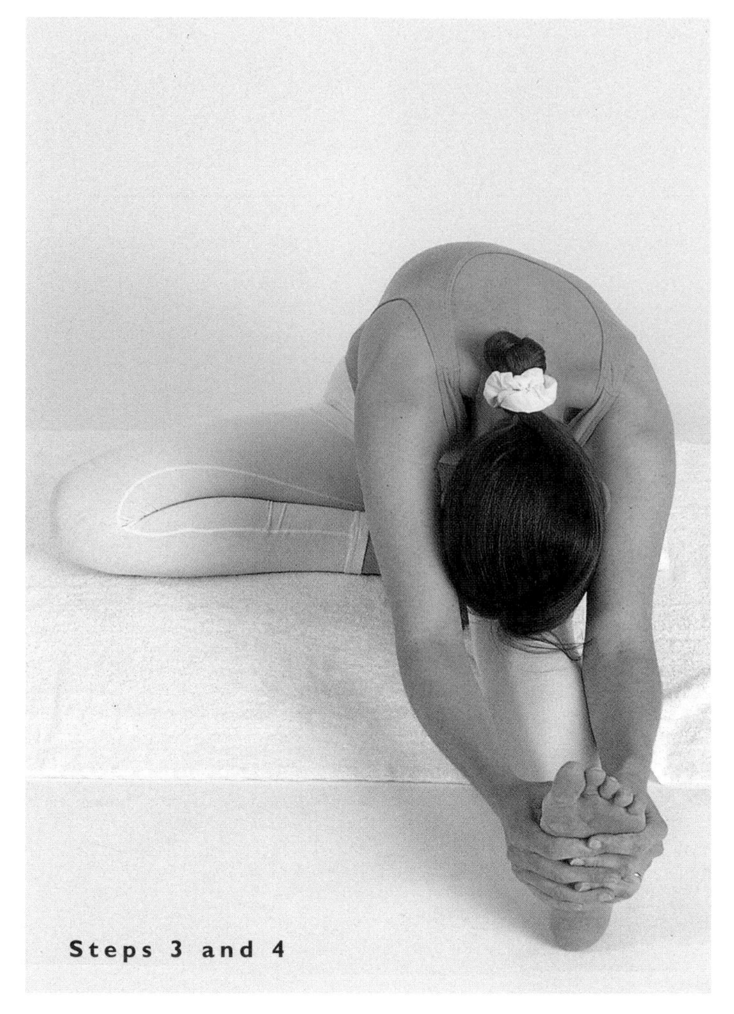

Steps 3 and 4

2. Place your hands just below the knee. At first keep your back straight as you begin to bend forward. Inhale. Bend from the hips — feel how you can pivot at the joints.

3. As you exhale, bend further forward and bring your head towards the knee. If you can, grasp your foot with your hands. Keep the hips down.

4. Hold, breathing normally, extending and loosening with each exhalation.

Sitting stretches loosen the pelvic region, elongate muscles and improve flexibility. Stretch a little more — gently and patiently — on each exhalation.

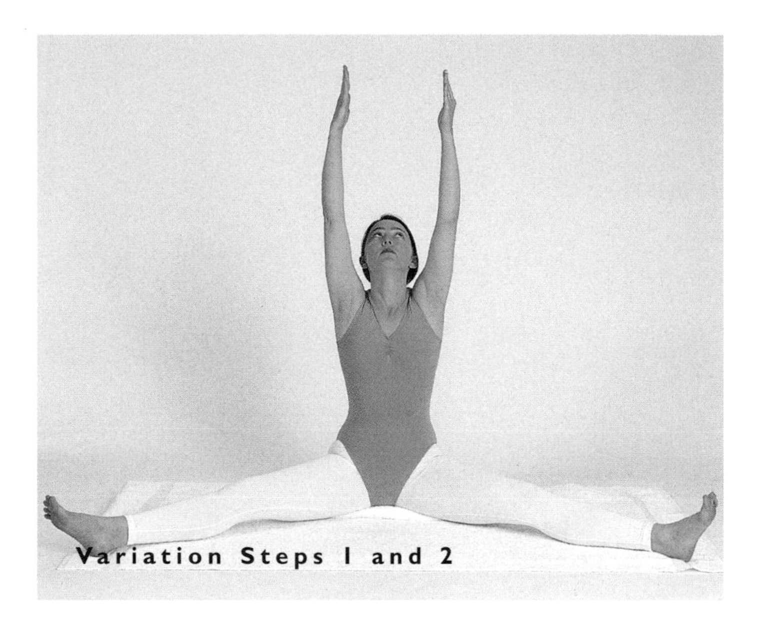
Variation Steps 1 and 2

Variation

This posture is known as a Wide Leg Stretch.

1. Sit with the legs wide apart.
2. Breathing in, stretch your arms above your head. Lengthen the spine as you reach for the ceiling.
3. Turn your body from the hips so you are facing your right leg.
4. As you breathe out, extend from the hips and reach down to touch your right foot with your hands. This should be one movement.
5. Inhale, and return to the center position (Step 2).
6. This time, as you exhale, bring your head towards the floor in front of you.
7. Return to the central position, then swivel and reach down your leg towards the left.
8. Continue the movement in this circular fashion. Always stretch upwards before stretching forwards and down. Remember to breathe in as you stretch up, and out as you stretch down. Sitting on a folded blanket or cushion will help you to bend from the hips, and relieve pressure on the tailbone.

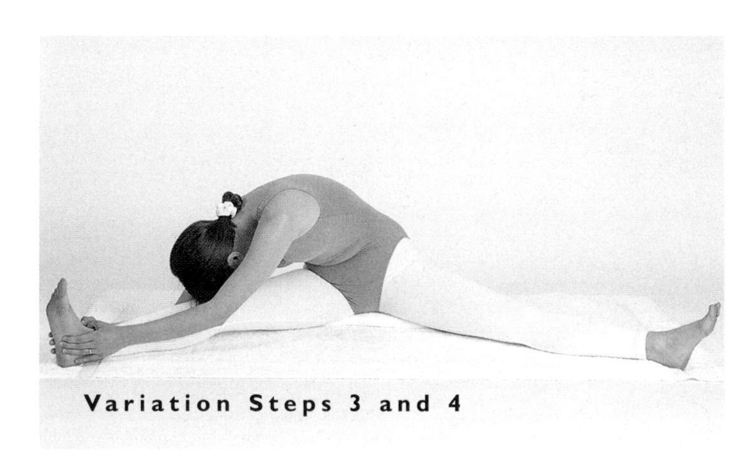
Variation Steps 3 and 4

Benefits

- stretches the hamstrings
- loosens the whole body
- increases flexibility at the hip joints
- massages the liver, spleen and kidneys
- tones the female reproductive system
- stimulates circulation
- soothes lower back pain

Caution

Do not strain — elongate gently and patiently. Avoid injuring the back or thigh muscles.

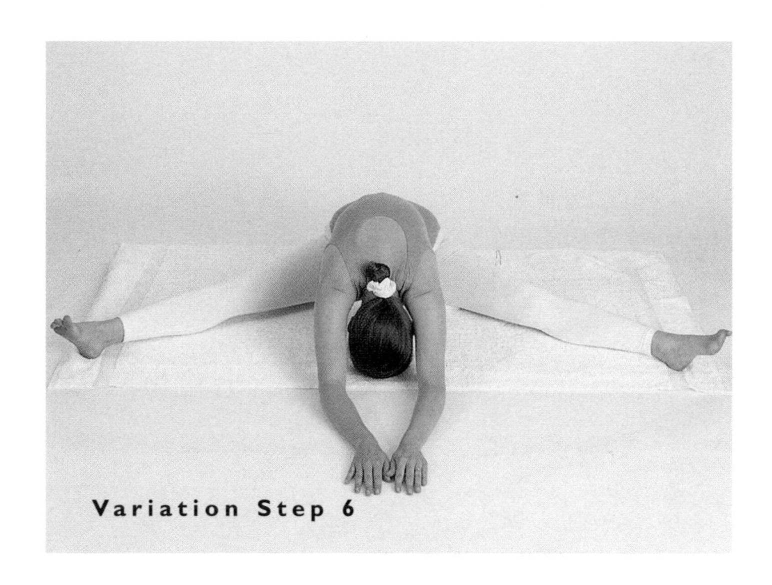
Variation Step 6

HALF-SPINAL TWIST

ARDHA MATSYENDRASANA

TWIST

The sitting twist postures feel wonderful, especially at the end of a long day, or even after a long sleep. Always try to include a twist after practicing forward and backward bends. This will significantly ease the back muscles. You may like to place a cushion or folded blanket beneath your buttocks for support.

When you feel compressed and sluggish, try a twist to realign your body, release tight muscles and activate stagnant energy.

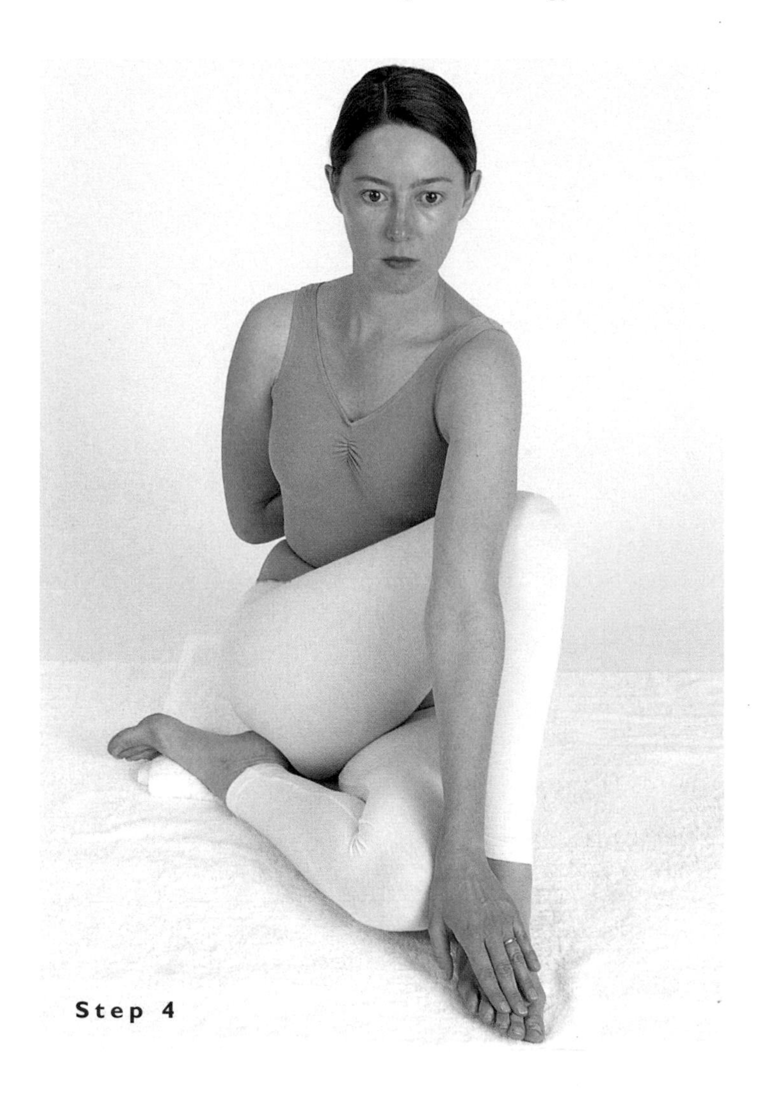

Step 4

1. Sit with your legs stretched in front of you.
2. Take the right foot and place it outside the left knee.
3. Bend the left leg so the foot rests as close as possible to your right buttock.
4. Hold the right ankle with your left hand. Make sure your arm is resting on the *outer side* of the raised leg. Make sure the knee is close to the armpit.
5. Fold the other arm behind your back, or rest it on the floor behind you. Inhale deeply. Now you are ready to twist.
6. Exhale, and slowly twist your body and your head towards the right. Feel tense muscles unwind. Remain in the position for a few seconds, breathing steadily. Keep looking towards the wall behind you.
7. On an exhalation, try twisting a little more but do not strain your body.
8. Inhale as you return to position 1, with your legs stretched in front. Repeat the twist to the other side.

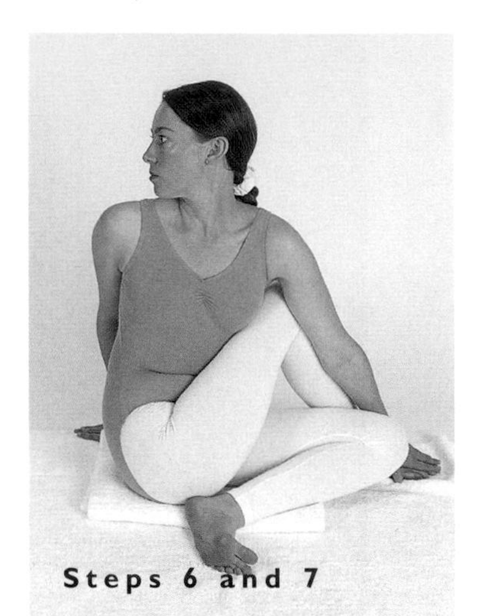

Steps 6 and 7

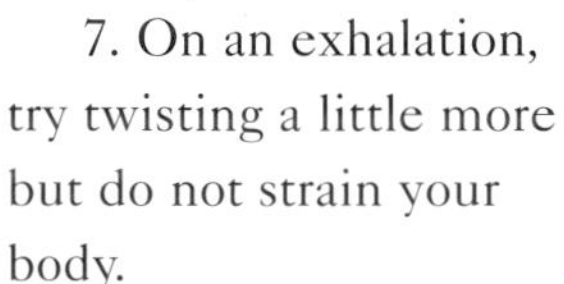

Awareness

Work into the posture. With every exhalation, release tension from your back. Twist, stop, lengthen the spine upwards, twist, stop, lengthen. At the end of the twist, see how your body feels stronger, straighter and longer.

Benefits

- releases back tension
- aligns and strengthens the spine
- increases flexibility
- stimulates the nervous system
- tones abdominal organs
- regulates the adrenal gland
- aids the function of the pancreas

Caution

Do not force the body — if you feel pain, you have twisted too far. If you have a back problem such as a displaced disc, only practice twists under the supervision of a teacher.

Floor postures

CORPSE AND REVERSED CORPSE

SAVASANA AND ADVASANA

REST

The Corpse and its reversed form are the resting poses for the floor exercises. However, you can lie in these postures at any time throughout a yoga session if you are feeling tired or need to slow the pulse. The Corpse pose is also used for the total relaxation practice (see page 59). See the variation on 'Hero' on page 33 as an alternative resting pose.

THE CORPSE

1. Lie on the floor on your back. Your feet should be a small distance apart, your arms resting comfortably at your sides. Face palms upwards.

2. Close your eyes. Let every muscle in your body soften and relax. Breathe deeply and slowly. Try to remain still and quiet.

THE REVERSED CORPSE

1. Lie on your stomach.

2. Part your legs a little, place arms by your sides, palms facing upwards.

3. Turn your head to one side. If you are remaining in the posture for some time, change the direction of your head occasionally.

Variation

The Reversed Corpse may be practiced with your arms stretched out in front of you and your forehead resting on the floor.

This posture is particularly suited to people with stiff necks and back problems. It also elongates the spine after bending poses.

Benefits

- relaxes the whole body
- balances the physiological processes of the body
- stills the mind and emotions
- promotes sleep

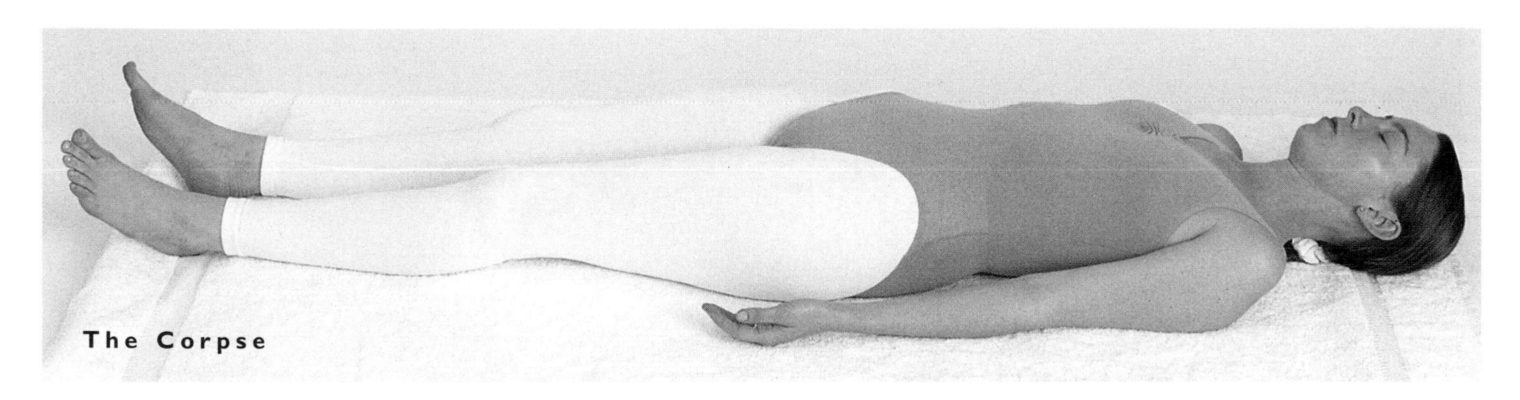

The Corpse

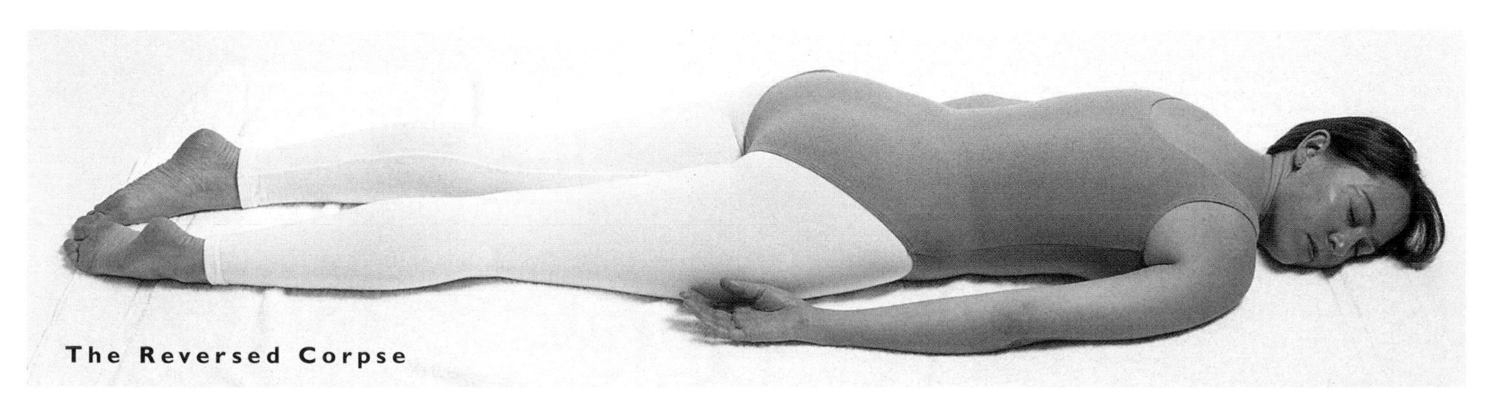

The Reversed Corpse

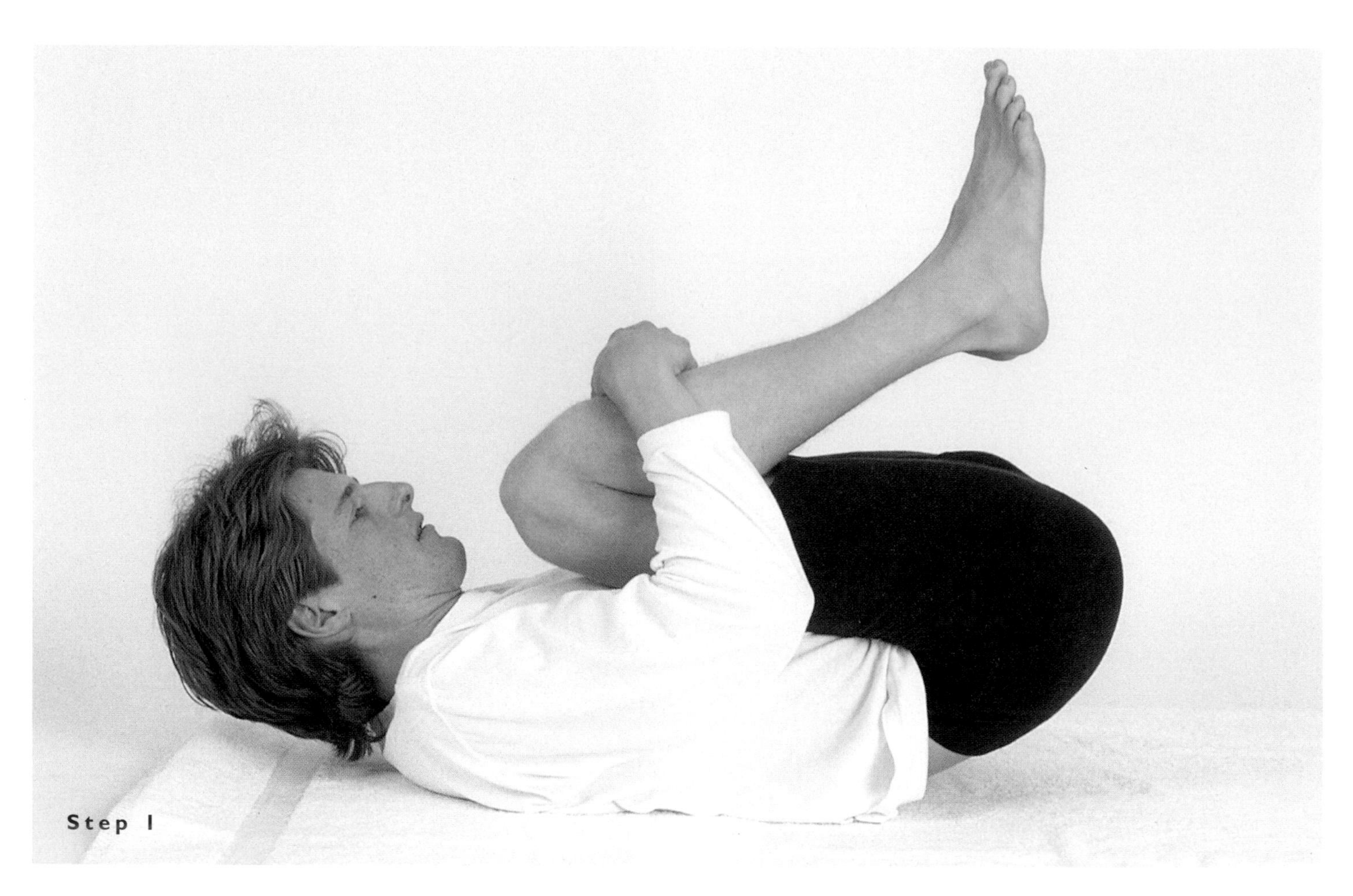

ROCKING AND ROLLING

LOOSENER

Rocking and Rolling is a fun posture which loosens and warms the whole body. Try this posture at the beginning of a yoga session or to get you moving in the morning.

1. Lie on your back and bring your knees to your chest. Clasp your arms around your knees.

2. Let your body roll gently backwards, then roll forwards, keeping your body in the curled position. When you roll forwards try to come into a squatting position.

3. Continue rocking and rolling backwards and forwards, creating one smooth movement.

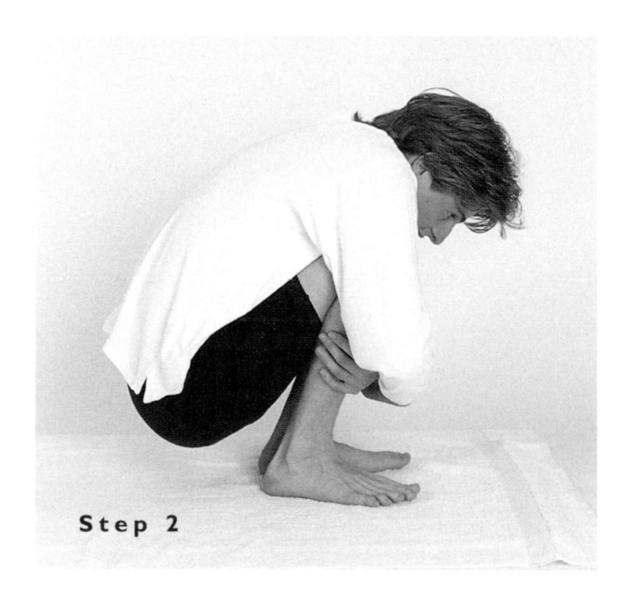

Benefits

- Stimulates energy flow in the body
- Massages the whole spine and back
- Warms the body before a yoga session

Caution

When you roll backwards be careful not to hit your head on the floor. Do not rock and roll on a hard surface. Make sure you have a mat or folded blanket beneath the spine.

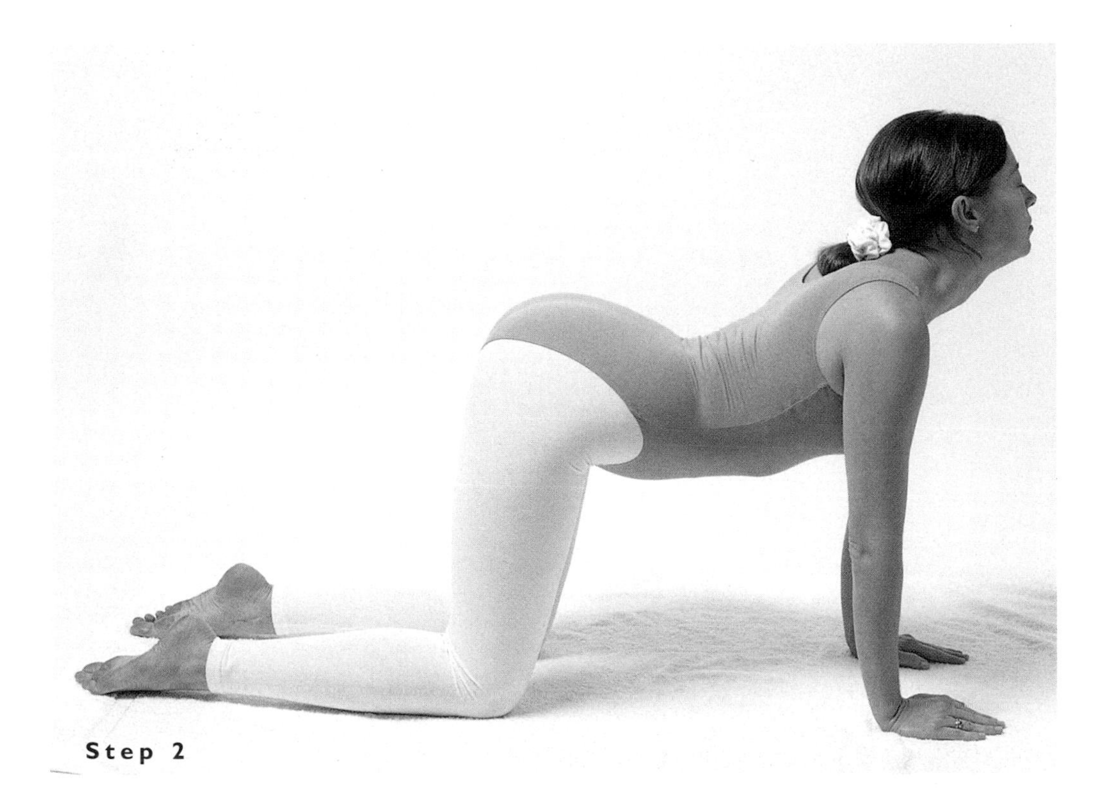

Step 2

The Cat pose gently loosens the whole spine. As you arch and curve your back, imagine yourself to be a cat, as she stretches after a long sleep.

CAT

MARJARIASANA

STRETCH

The Cat stretch is one of the most relaxing of all the yoga poses. It loosens and stretches the entire spinal column. An excellent posture if you have been sitting at a desk all day.

1. Kneel so that your hands rest directly below your shoulders, your knees below your hips. Hold your head in line with the spine. Check that your legs and arms are parallel to each other.
2. Inhale, and arch your back. Expand your chest and let your neck curve backwards. Keep your arms straight. Hold.
3. As you exhale, let your head lower towards your chest and curve your back.
4. Continue in a flowing motion to curve and arch your back. Observe the increased sense of space between the vertebrae of your spine.

Awareness

The use of the breath is very important in the Cat stretch. Always breathe in deeply as you arch your back, and exhale fully as you curve your back. Keep the breath even.

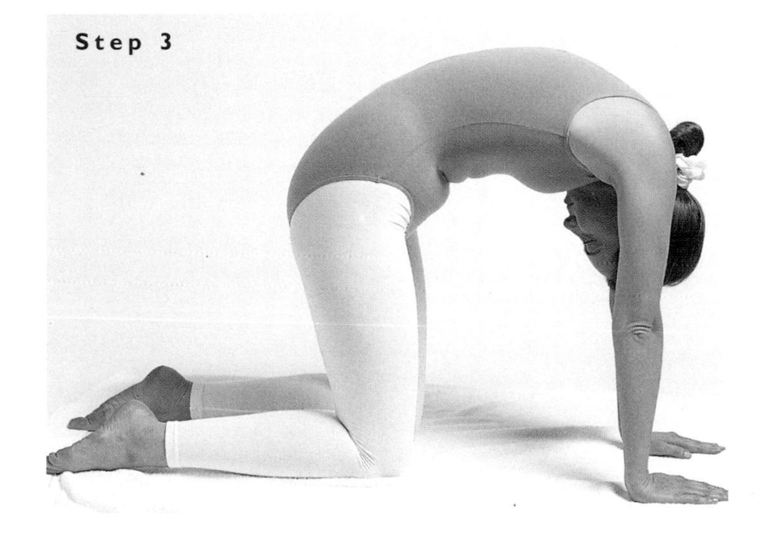

Step 3

Be aware of the spine from the very base to the top of the neck. Close your eyes and "experience" the posture. Feel your back lengthening and loosening as you stretch.

Benefits

- Stretches and loosens the spine
- Improves flexibility and posture
- Tones the reproductive system
- Eases menstrual pain
- Relieves constipation
- Firms the buttocks and thighs

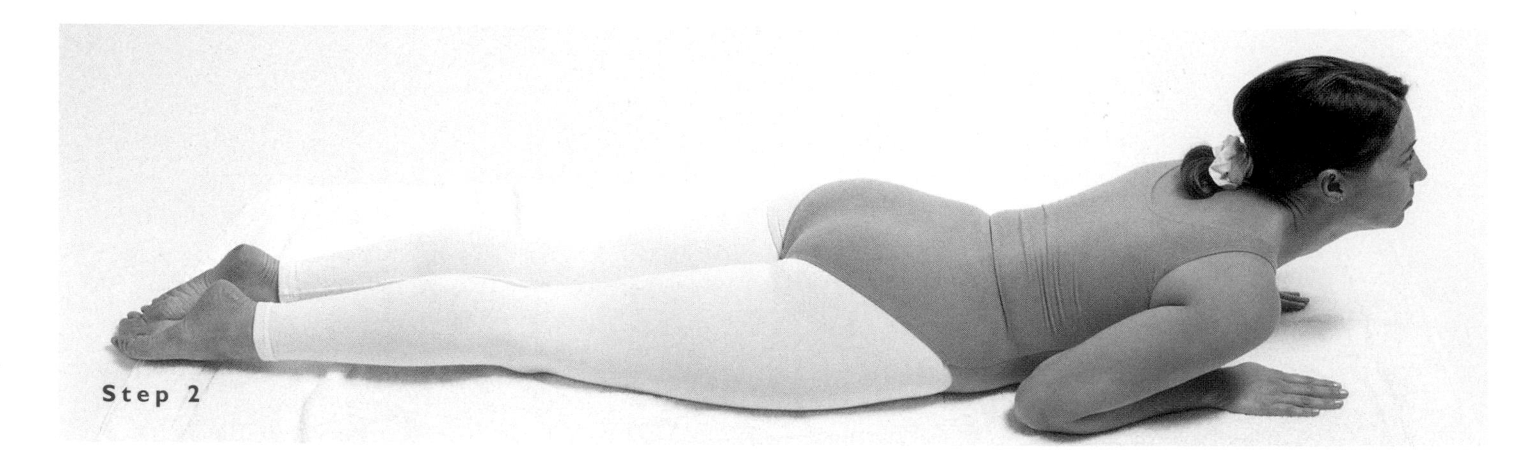

COBRA

BHUJANGASANA

BACKWARD BEND

The backward bend of the Cobra develops a supple spine and promotes good health. The muscles contract as you bend your back; then as you release the posture toxins are expelled and energy flows more freely.

1. Lie on your stomach and place your hands beneath your shoulders. Place palms flat on the floor, fingers facing forward, elbows close to your body. Legs and feet should be held together. Rest your forehead on the floor.

2. As you inhale, begin to raise your head from the floor. Once your head is a few inches from the floor, begin to raise your shoulders.

3. Continue to lift your chest and lengthen your arms. Keep your hips on the floor. Stretch forward so your chest is reaching towards the front wall. At this stage the arms are still bent at the elbow, and your head is facing forward.

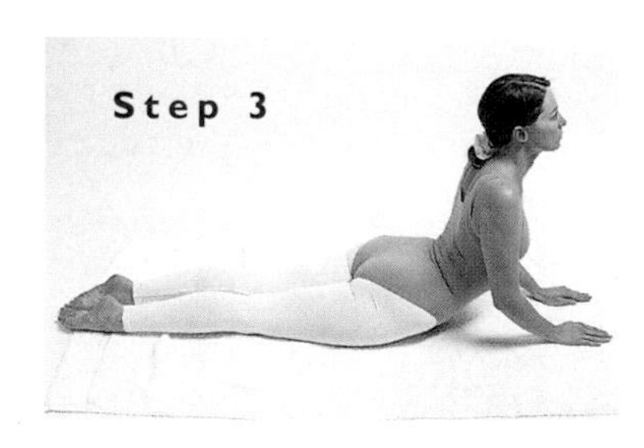

4. If you can straighten your arms without strain, do so. Let your neck arch backwards and look toward the ceiling. If you feel a pinching in your back do not straighten your arms.

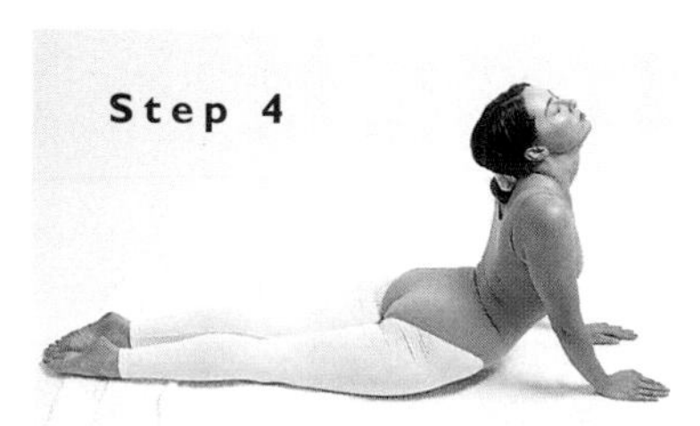

5. As you exhale, lower your body to the floor. Do this in reverse order — that is, lower your chest first, then shoulders and lastly bring your forehead to the floor. You will feel the vertebrae lowering one by one.

6. Rest in the Reversed Corpse pose (see page 41).

Awareness

As you practice this posture, keep in mind the image of a cobra. This snake can rear the front half of its body while its back half rests on the ground. Each vertebrae is raised then lowered in turn. It is essential to keep your hips on the floor and your navel reaching towards the floor. Open your chest and keep your legs together. Use your back muscles to raise the spine — do not push back with your arms.

Benefits

- Strengthens the spine
- Relieves backache
- Fortifies bladder function
- Regulates the menstrual cycle
- Helps constipation
- Tones abdominal organs
- Improves the appetite
- Flushes out stored toxins
- Provides a fresh blood flow to the spine

Caution

Practice the Cobra with patience. Do not stretch further than is comfortable. You should not experience any pain. Instead, extend the practice gently — increase the backward bend just a little with each attempt. Do not practice the Cobra if you have a peptic ulcer, hyper-thyroidism, a hernia or have recently undergone any kind of abdominal surgery. Avoid during menstruation. Take care if you have high blood pressure.

DOG

SVANASANA

FORWARD BEND/STRETCH

A dog gets up after a rest and slowly stretches. He pushes his rear toward the sky, his head to the ground and elongates the whole spine. This is Svanasana.

The Dog pose is very invigorating — it lengthens the spine, stretches the hamstrings and redirects blood to the brain. After practicing the Dog, you will suddenly feel much taller.

1. Kneel on "all fours" as in position 1 of the Cat stretch (see page 43). Make sure your body is aligned — your hands and feet should form four corners of a long rectangle.
2. Inhale and tuck your toes under, lifting your heels from the floor.
3. Exhale, and raise your buttocks toward the ceiling, straightening your legs. Lengthen your arms until the spine is in one line from the base to the nape of the neck. You will feel a stretch in the hamstrings behind the knees.
4. Keeping the buttocks high, lower your heels so your feet are flat on the floor. Let your head be loose and free, hanging between your arms.
5. Breathe normally in this position for as long as is comfortable.
6. Exhale, and lower the knees to the floor, then rest in the Child pose (see page 34).

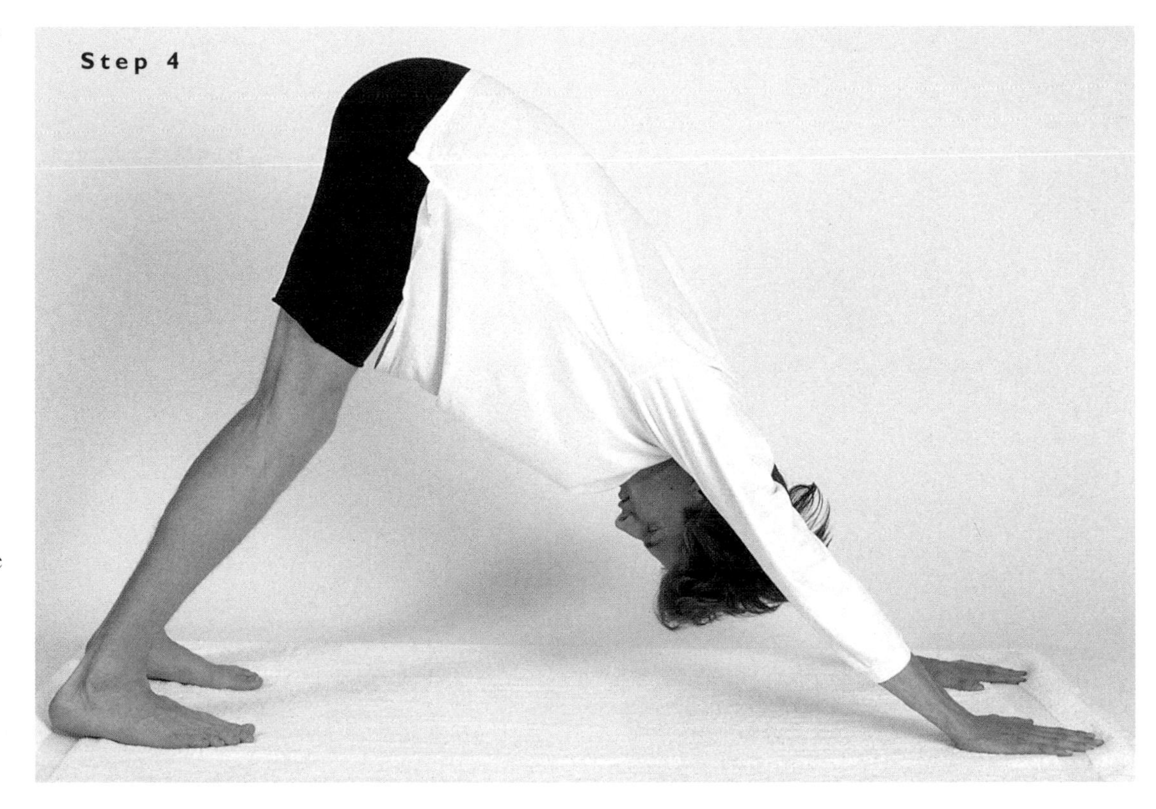

Step 4

Awareness

Concentrate on pushing your buttocks high, lengthening the spine from its base. Open your chest. Pull your abdomen in. Let the legs stretch up and back. The hip is the pivotal point — the legs stretch up to this point, while the upper torso stretches down from it. The body should form two sides of a triangle.

A good way to practice this posture is to have a partner place their hands on the base of your spine and apply gentle pressure pushing downwards toward your head. You will feel the lower vertebrae open and lengthen.

Benefits

- stretches the spinal column
- opens the chest — encourages deeper breathing
- strengthens the shoulders, arms and legs
- elongates the hamstrings
- stimulates the spinal nerves
- reduces the workload of the heart
- invigorates the whole body

Caution

Do not remain in the Dog pose for long periods if you are prone to high blood pressure. Do not practice after abdominal operations. Avoid during menstruation.

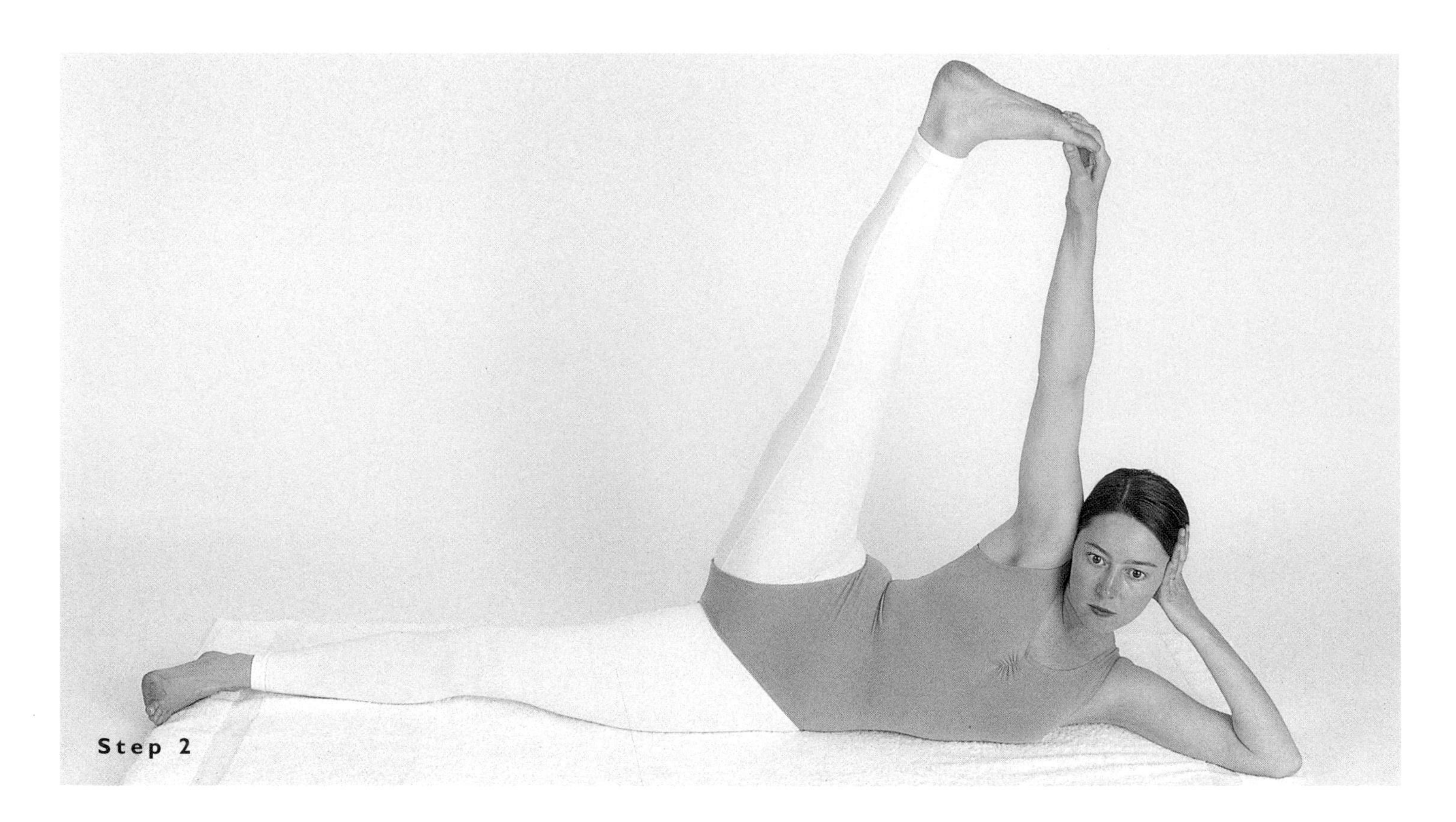

INFINITE STRETCH

ANANTASANA

STRETCH

The Infinite pose gives a full stretch to the whole leg. This posture is quite restful and can be used at the beginning or end of a yoga session to gently elongate calf and thigh muscles. After practicing the Dog pose (see page 45), the Infinite pose will calm the hamstrings.

1. Lie on the floor on your left side. Your left leg is on the floor, while the right leg is resting on top of the left. Bend your left elbow so your head is well supported by your hand. Your body is in one straight line.

2. Inhale, and slowly begin to raise your right leg. At the same time, slide your right hand up the leg. Grasp the toes with your hand. Both leg and arm should be straight. Breathe normally as you hold the position. Try to keep your body balanced on the side — do not roll backwards onto your buttocks. Move your weight forwards and backwards to find the position you feel most stable.

3. Exhale, lowering your arm and leg. Repeat to the other side.

Variation

Try this simple practice to stretch the hamstrings and improve flexibility at the hips. Lie on your back with legs together. Raise your legs into the air and place a rope around both feet. Hold the rope with your hands, and very gently draw your legs towards your head. Relax, then pull your legs a little closer. Keep hips on the floor.

A rope can be used in this way to enhance most of the stretching postures.

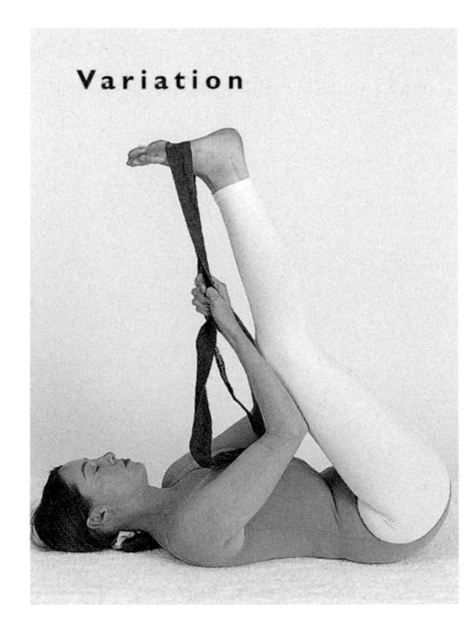

Benefits

- gently stretches the legs
- tones the thigh muscles, reducing fat deposits
- soothes the hamstrings
- opens the pelvis
- relieves backache
- massages the abdominal muscles

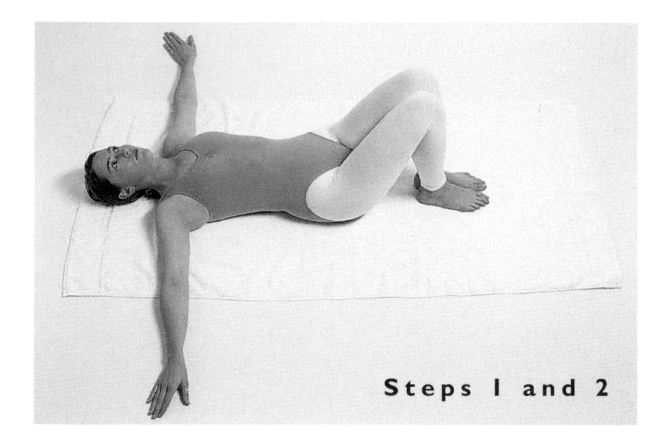

Steps 1 and 2

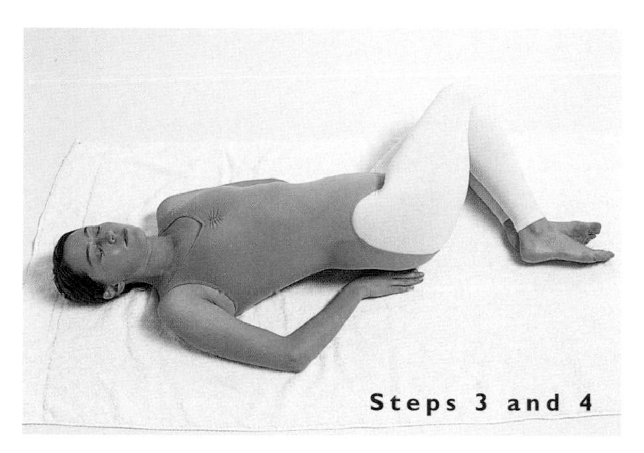

Steps 3 and 4

SUPINE TWIST

JATHARA PARIVARTASANA

TWIST

Twists performed on the floor are restful and help to ease lower back pain. Work gently, letting your body relax and stretch into the posture — avoid any strain.

1. Lie on your back, arms stretched out at shoulder height. Make sure the arms form a straight line. Alternately, you can place your hands palms down underneath your buttocks for support.
2. Bend your knees and place feet flat on the floor.
3. Inhale. As you exhale move your knees towards the floor on the left hand side. Turn your head to the right and gaze towards your fingertips. Feel the opening of your lower back. Only drop the knees as far as is comfortable — they need not reach the floor.
4. Breathe normally and completely relax your body.
5. Inhale, and raise your legs to the center again.
6. Exhale, and move your legs to the right, and your head to the left. Continue twisting slowly in this manner.

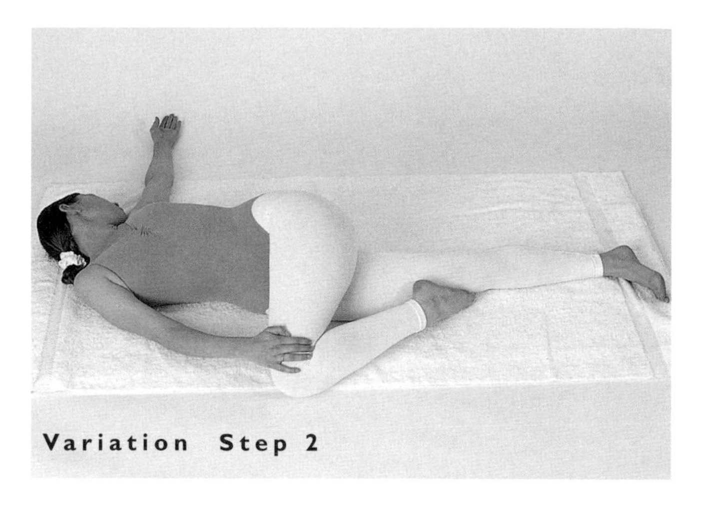

Variation Step 2

Variation

For a stronger twist, try this variation:

1. Lie on the floor, this time keeping your right leg straight. Bend your left leg and place it across the right, so the foot rests on the outer side of the knee. Stretch your left arm out at shoulder height and rest your right hand on the right knee.
2. As you exhale, twist so the bent knee reaches to the right, across the straight leg, to the floor. Look towards the left. Try to keep your left shoulder on the floor — you will feel the stretch this gives. Use your hand to gently push your leg towards the floor.
3. Return to center position, and lower your left leg to the floor. Now, bend your right leg and repeat the twist to the other side.

Awareness

As you rest in these twists, observe the areas of your body which are storing tension. With every exhalation, let this tension go — you do not need it. Feel all the muscles unwind, your body gently realign, and sense a fresh supply of blood flow to all the abdominal organs. Notice how alive your body feels at the end of these practices.

Benefits

- eases lower back pain
- aligns the spine
- stretches waist, hip, shoulder and neck muscles
- reduces tension in the body
- massages the abdominal organs
- increases flexibility

Inverted postures

The inverted postures are very rejuvenating and rid the body of all lethargy. They are quite restful, and help to pacify anxiety and intense emotion.

Caution

• Care should be taken in all inverted postures.
• Work slowly and gently.
• Do not hold postures for too long at first.
• If you feel any strain or pressure in the neck, back, head, ears, eyes or throat, come down and rest in the Child pose (see page 34).
• Avoid inverted postures if you have any of the following conditions:
– high blood pressure
– heart problems
– eye or ear problems
– enlarged thyroid or spleen
– a chronic illness (seek advice)
• Cease the practice of inverted postures during menstruation.

If you have a neck or back injury, practice under the supervision of a teacher. When you are putting weight on the neck, it is easily injured.

WALL STAND

INVERTED REST

The Wall Stand is a gentle inverted posture,in which you can rest for long periods. Try a Wall Stand to ease the legs after a hard day. You may like to rest with the legs together or wide apart — whichever you find most soothing. Try covering your eyes with a soft cloth to enhance the effect.

1. Lie on the floor with your buttocks against a wall. You may need to curl up on your side, then swivel to get your buttocks close to the wall.
2. Stretch your legs so they are straight up and resting on the wall. Close your eyes and rest peacefully.
3. Now, gently widen the legs to a comfortable distance.
4. Relax and breathe deeply.

Benefits

• restores flagging energy
• soothes tired legs
• relieves headache
• calms the mind and emotions

In the inverted postures all is reversed.
Restful and relaxing, these postures restore energy and calm the mind.
The legs are relieved of their duties, blood flows to the brain
and the whole body comes alive.

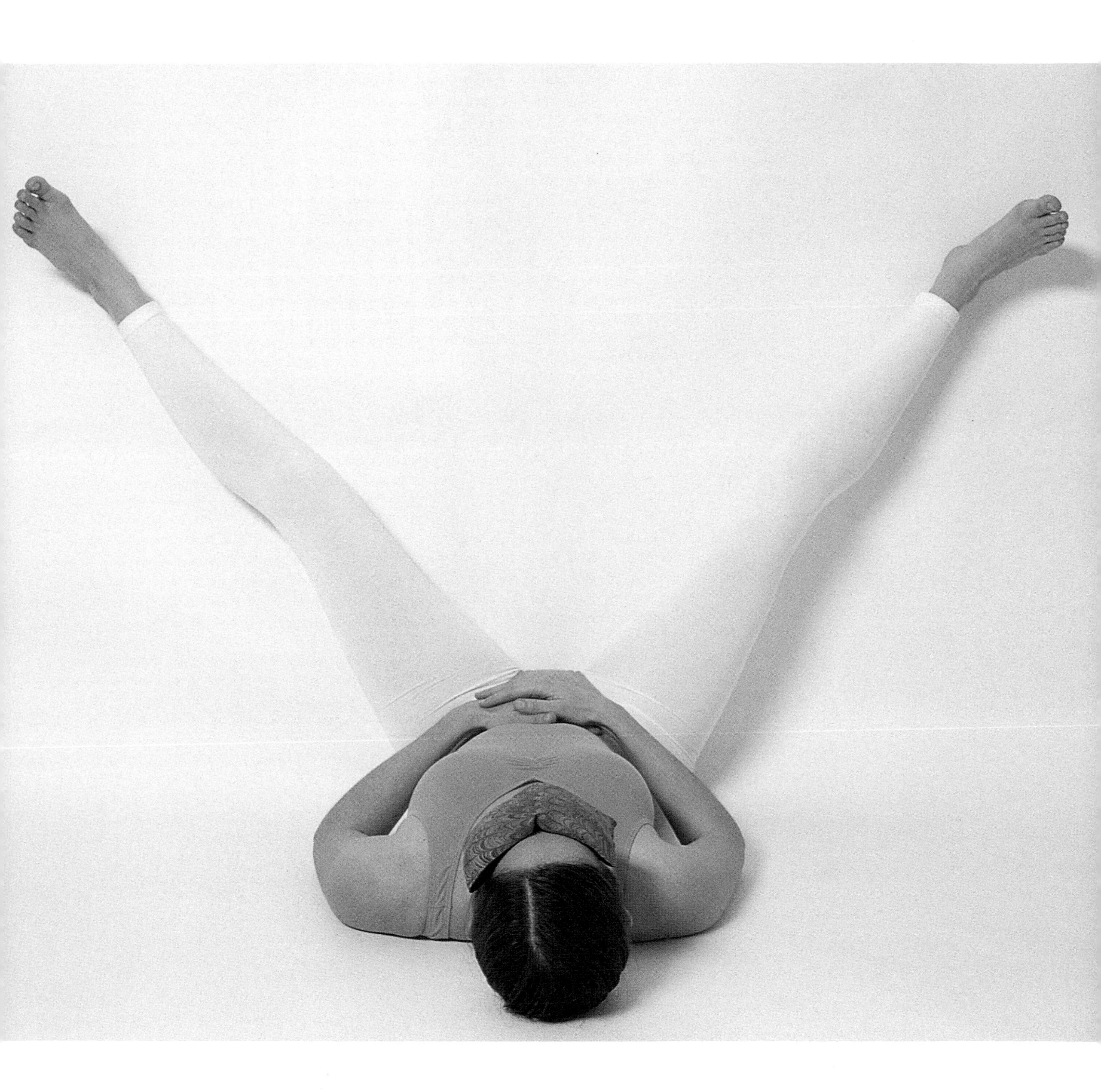

SHOULDER STAND

SARVANGASANA

INVERTED

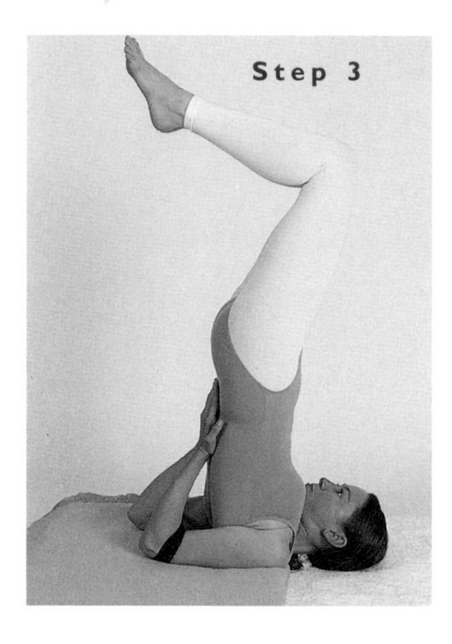

The Shoulder Stand is a classic inverted posture. It nourishes the whole body and stimulates the thyroid gland, located at the base of the neck. However, the posture is only of benefit if practiced with care. It is very important not to strain the neck.

1. Place one or two neatly folded blankets on the floor.
2. Lie on your back on the blanket so your shoulders and arms are on the blanket, but your head is resting on the floor. Rest your arms beside your body and then inhale.
3. As you exhale, slowly begin to raise your legs from the floor, bending them as they lift upwards. At the same time place your hands on your back for support. Try to keep the elbows inward and parallel. If this is difficult, place a belt around them before beginning the practice. You may need someone to help you with this.
4. Once you are steady and balanced, raise your legs to a straight position. Push your chest towards your chin. Use your hands to help your body form one straight line.
5. Hold for a few seconds, breathing steadily.
6. Exhale and come out of the posture by bending the legs and gently unrolling onto the floor.
7. Rest in the Child pose, with arms extended (see page 34).

Variation

If you find the Shoulder Stand difficult, try:

- Practicing only up to step 3, to begin with.
- Practicing the posture supported by a wall. Lie with your buttocks close to the wall and bend your legs so your feet are resting flat on the wall. Push up onto your shoulders from this position. Make sure you have a folded blanket beneath your shoulders.

Benefits

- delivers a fresh flow of blood to the brain
- stimulates the thyroid gland, which in turn balances the metabolism of the whole body
- aids respiratory problems
- tones the legs and trims the waist
- wards off varicose veins
- strengthens the reproductive and urinary organs
- helps to overcome emotional problems such as anxiety and depression
- refreshes and sharpens the mind
- restores vitality to the body

Caution

Do not move your head once you have commenced the posture. This can cause damage to the neck. If you feel your neck is not straight, come down and begin again. If you experience any pain or compression in the neck, or a sense of dizziness, cease the practice and rest. Always remember to keep your face and throat relaxed.

Avoid the practice if you have high blood pressure, spinal injury or are menstruating.

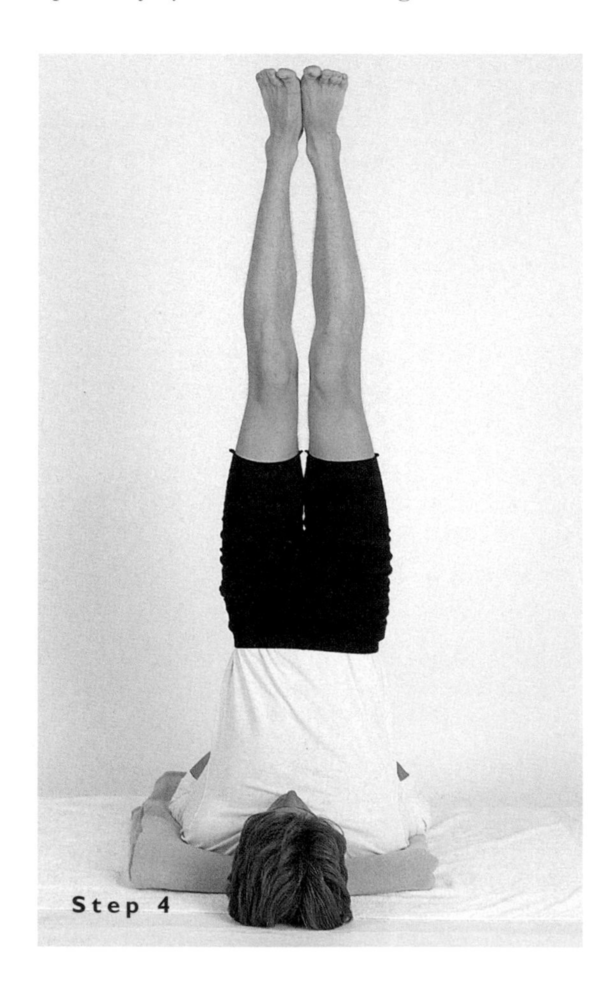

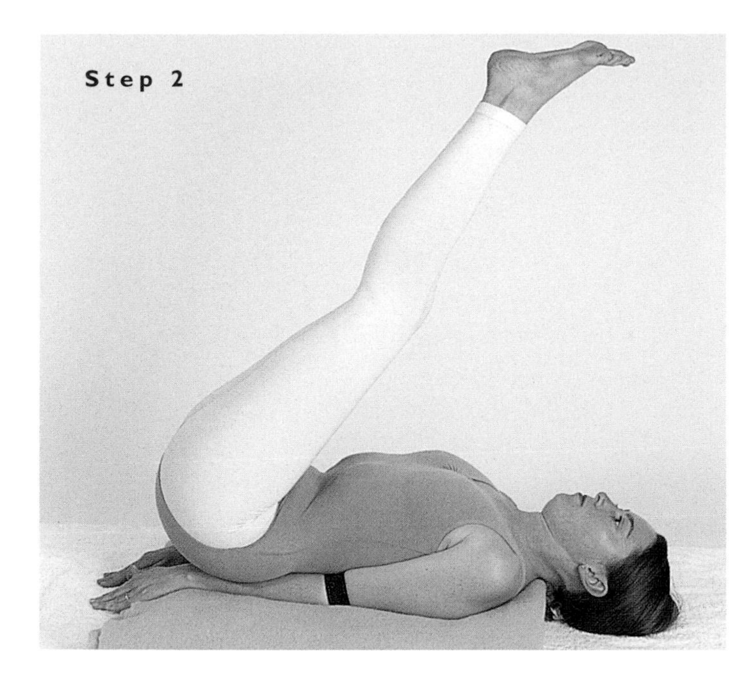
Step 2

PLOUGH
HALASANA

INVERTED

The Plough is quite a strong practice but is excellent for all the internal organs. The Plough follows naturally from the Shoulder Stand.

1. Lie on the floor, resting the shoulders on folded blankets as in the Shoulder Stand, position 1 (see opposite). Inhale. Place your hands at your side, palms down.

2. As you exhale, begin to lift both legs from the floor, holding them close together.

3. As you raise your legs, start to bend your torso upwards, hips leading. Immediately support your back with your hands. Your chest should be moving closer to your chin. Push your buttocks toward the ceiling and bring your legs over your head, so the toes are touching the floor behind you. Straighten your legs if you can. If this is difficult, you can bend them. Remember, always work at your own pace. In yoga practice, there is no hurry or pressure to perform.

4. Breathe normally and hold for a short time.

5. On an exhalation, slowly uncurl your body, vertebrae by vertebrae, onto the floor. It is beneficial to rest in Supta Virasana (see page 33) after the Plough posture.

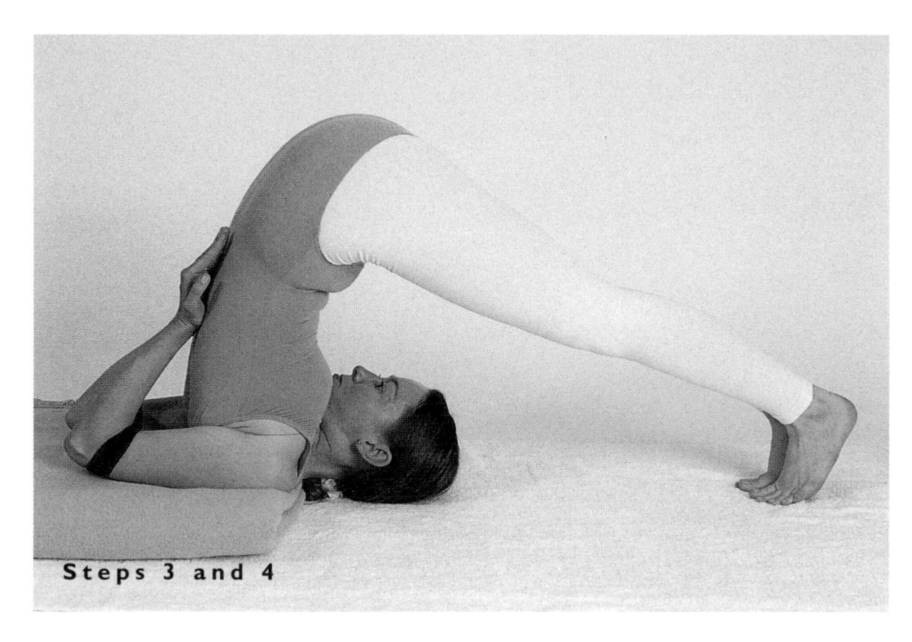
Steps 3 and 4

Variation
It is possible to lower into the Plough from the Shoulder Stand. Once you are well balanced in the vertical position of the Shoulder Stand, gently lower the toes to the floor behind you.

Awareness
Press your chest forward with your hands.

Keep elbows in (use a belt if required). When you raise your legs, concentrate on using the abdominal muscles, not your arms — they are for support only. As you hold the posture, close your eyes and feel your body rejuvenating.

Benefits
- stimulates the digestive organs
- balances the functioning of the liver, pancreas and kidneys
- stimulates the thyroid, parathyroid, pineal and pituitary glands
- encourages blood flow to the brain
- massages and opens the spine
- relieves constipation
- rejuvenates the cells of the body
- sharpens and calms the mind

Caution
As with the Shoulder Stand — do not practice the posture if you are feeling discomfort — consult a teacher. Avoid the Plough if you have any back injury, sciatica, high blood pressure or during menstruation.

Salute to the Sun

SURYA NAMASKAR

Surya Namaskar brings life to every cell.
When the energy levels have dwindled, just one or two
rounds of Salute will revive the whole being.

Salute to the Sun is a practice composed of 12 successive steps. These 12 positions flow together into one long movement.

Salute to the Sun massages every part of the body — it is a full exercise regime in itself. The muscles, the internal organs, the body systems and the brain are all stimulated. Practice the Salute first thing in the morning to welcome the new day.

1. Stand tall with the feet slightly apart and the hands in a prayer position at the level of the heart. Relax your body, breathing steadily.

2. Inhale, raising your arms above your head. Hold the arms shoulder width apart and turn the palms to the sky. Bend your head and upper torso backwards slightly, opening your chest.

3. Exhale, and bend forward from the hips, reaching towards the floor with your hands. If you can do so, place your hands flat on the floor — but make sure you are not straining any part of the body.

4. Inhale, and stretch your right foot backwards, lowering the knee to the floor. Raise the heel of your right foot, tucking the toes under. Simultaneously bend your left knee. Keep your arms straight and move the hips towards the floor. Tilt your head slightly backwards and gaze upwards.

5. Exhale, and push your buttocks towards the sky, taking your left foot back to meet the right. Both legs should be straight, the arms straight and your head hanging loosely between your arms. Your body forms two sides of a triangle. Lengthen the spine from the base. (See the Dog pose, page 45).

6. Holding the breath, bring your knees to the floor. Push your buttocks backwards and upwards so you can slide your chest along the ground. Push your upper torso forward between your arms. Hold your elbows close to your body.

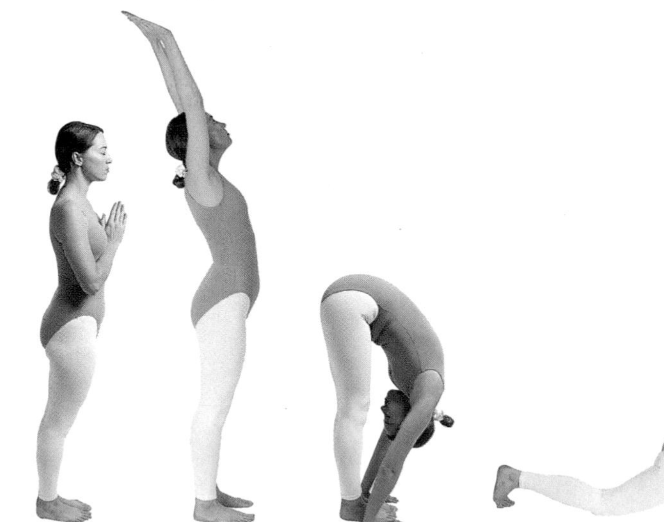

Step 1 Step 2 Step 3 Step 4

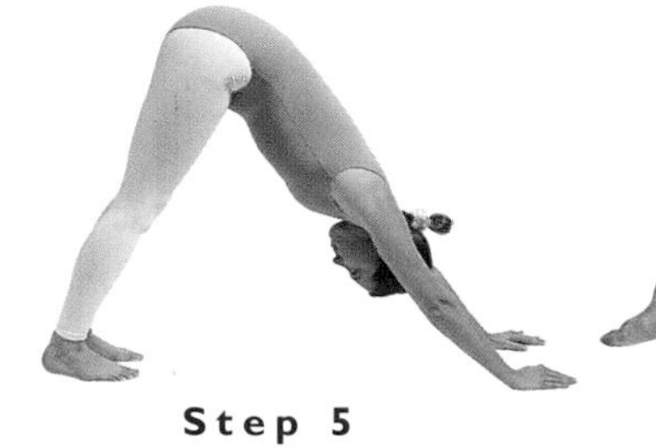

Step 5

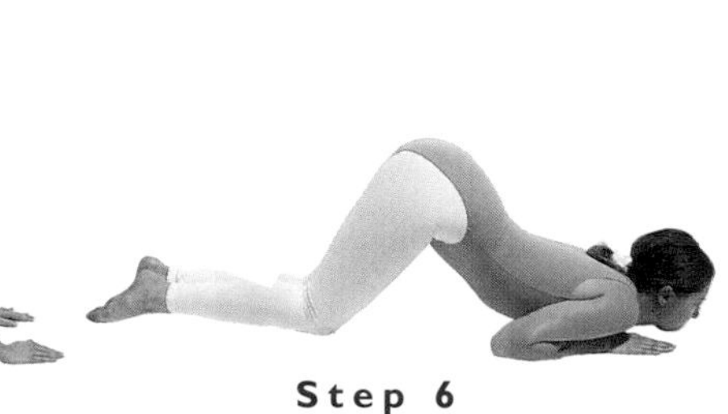

Step 6

Surya Namaskar is an ancient Indian practice which is traditionally done before sunrise. Practice the Salute in the morning, synchronizing all movements with inhalations and exhalations, for a great start to the day.

7. Inhale, and continue to slide your body forwards, lowering the hips onto the floor and raising your upper torso from the waist. You may straighten your arms or keep them bent, whichever suits your own body. Tilt your head backwards slightly and gaze towards the sky. (See the Cobra pose, page 44).

8. Exhaling, raise your buttocks in the air and return to step 5, the Dog pose.

9. Inhale, and stretch your right leg back, bending the left – as in step 4.

10. Exhale, and bring your right foot forward to the left, straightening both legs. Lower your head towards your knees and lower your hands towards the floor. See step 3.

11. Inhale, and float your arms above your head, arching backwards, as in step 2.

12. Exhale, and finally bring your hands to a prayer position once again. You have now returned to step 1.

Salute to the Sun is cyclic in design. From step 7, we return to step 1 by repeating steps 5 to 1 in reverse order.

Rest in the Corpse pose after completing the practice (see page 41). You may need to rest for some time before the heart slows and your body returns to normal.

This cycle of 12 steps constitutes half a round of Salute to the Sun. To complete a full round, repeat the whole practice, but this time stretch back with the left leg instead of the right in steps 4 and 9. Always finish the practice after a full round, so your body is balanced.

You can practice as many rounds of Surya Namaskar as desired. Depending on how your body feels at the time, you may choose to move from one step to the next very slowly, or quite dynamically. Experiment to see which pace is right for you.

Awareness

Concentrate on the breath. Salute to the Sun is a wave of stretching backwards and bending forwards postures. Notice how the correct use of the breath gives a smooth continuity to the practice. Breathe in fully as you stretch and breathe out as you bend. Feel fresh air filling your body, stale air leaving.

Caution

Do not overexert yourself in this practice. Salute to the Sun is very powerful. If you begin to feel weak or dizzy, cease the practice and rest. It may be you have released too many toxins into your body at once.

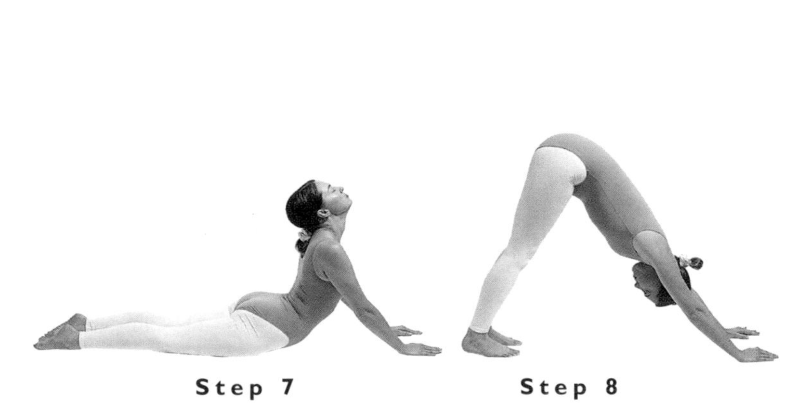

Step 7 **Step 8**

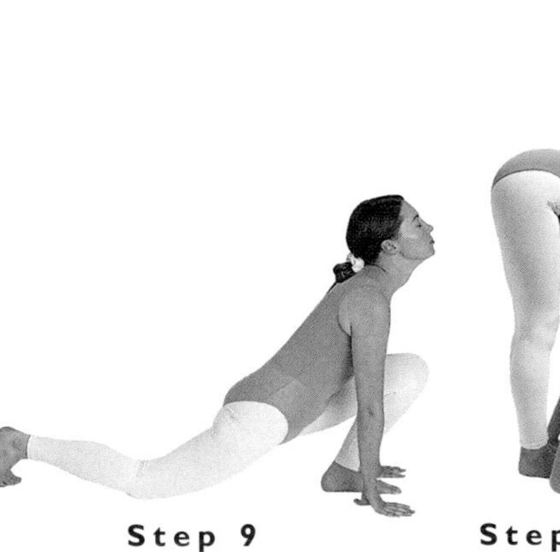

Step 9

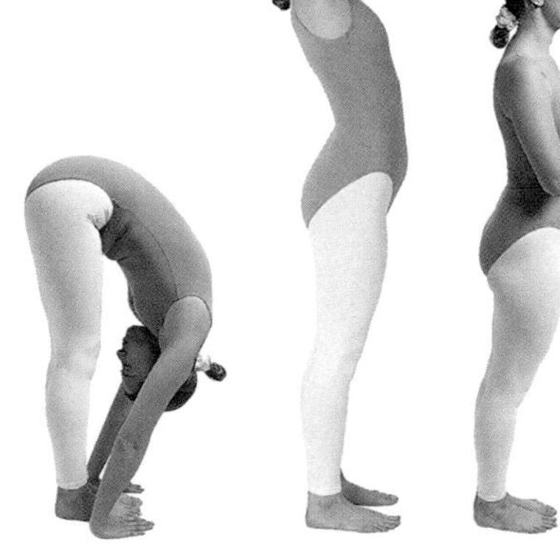

Step 10 **Step 11** **Step 12**

The Breath of Life

PRANAYAMA

Prana is vital energy. Yama is control.
With the subtle use of breath, tap into the vitality
which flows through you and all existence.

Breathing exercises help you to understand and control the essential energy or life force which fires all beings. With each breath, we bring fresh prana into the body. Stagnant energy is expelled with each exhalation. Breathe in the good, breathe out the bad.

Pranayama is invaluable in times of stress. The rhythmic motion of the breath subdues anxiety and composes the emotions. Most importantly, notice how clear the mind feels after these practices. Pranayama is an excellent way to sharpen the intellect.

How to sit

It is important to be comfortable and relaxed during Pranayama. Try the following postures:

- Easy cross-legged: Sit on the floor and fold your legs into a comfortable position.
- Half-Lotus: From the cross-legged position, take one foot and place it on the opposite thigh. Let your other foot rest on the floor. (See Humming Bee Breath pose on page 56).
- Full Lotus: Sit in the Half-Lotus position. Take the foot which is on the floor and lift it up and over the opposite leg, placing it on the opposite thigh. Now each foot is resting on the opposite thigh. The soles of the feet face upwards.

However you choose to sit, make certain the spine is straight and elongated. Your head should be in line with your spine and tilted slightly forward. Rest your hands on your knees or in your lap. Place a cushion or folded blanket beneath your buttocks. Close your eyes. If you find keeping your back straight difficult, use a wall for support.

Yogic breath

Most of us do not breathe to our full potential — we tend to "shallow breathe", which utilizes only a small percentage of the lung's capacity.

A full breath will transport much more oxygen into the blood, which fuels our energy. The yogic breath is also a wonderful way to relax. Place your hands, fingers interlaced, on each region as it fills with air. Notice how your fingers move apart as you inhale and come together as you exhale. The Yogic Breath may also be practiced in the Corpse position (see page 41).

1. *Breathe in* through your nose, directing the air to the abdomen only. Let the air completely fill the abdomen. Feel your abdomen swell. *Exhale.*

2. *Inhale,* and this time expand the rib cage area. The ribs will move outwards as you breathe. Inflate the lower lungs. The abdomen remains still. *Exhale,* and let the ribs move inwards.

3. Finally, *breathe in* and guide the air to the shoulder region. Fill the upper lungs with air, and allow the shoulders to expand.

4. Now, try combining steps 1 to 3 to create one long breath. Breathe in, filling the abdomen first, then the rib cage and finally the shoulder region. Exhale in the reverse order. First the shoulders, then the rib cage and finally the abdomen. Imagine the breath as one continuous, flowing wave. Saturate yourself with air.

ALTERNATE NOSTRIL BREATH

NADI SHODHAN PRANAYAMA

This is a very tranquil practice. It rids the body of toxins, balances the flow of energy and expels stale air. The brain cells are enlivened. It is important to keep the inhalation and exhalation the same length. Try counting: one, two, three, one, two, three ...

You may notice one nostril is more blocked than the other. This is usually the case. The practice of Nadi Shodhan ensures each nostril gets a turn – this is very important as breathing predominantly through one side can lead to disharmony in the body.

1. Using your right hand, place index and middle fingers on your brow, centered between your eyes. Let your thumb rest beside your right nostril, and your ring finger beside your left nostril.

2. Block the right nostril with your thumb and inhale through the left nostril. Draw the breath up towards the center of your eyebrows. Make the breath slow and even.

3. Now, block off the left nostril with your ring finger and exhale through the right.

4. Once all the air is expelled, inhale through the right nostril, keeping the left nostril blocked.

5. This time exhale through the left nostril, blocking the right.

6. Continue the practice, breathing in through one nostril and out the other. As you practice, see if you can lengthen the time of each breath in and out. However, never let yourself become out of breath. If you experience any discomfort, cease the practice and rest.

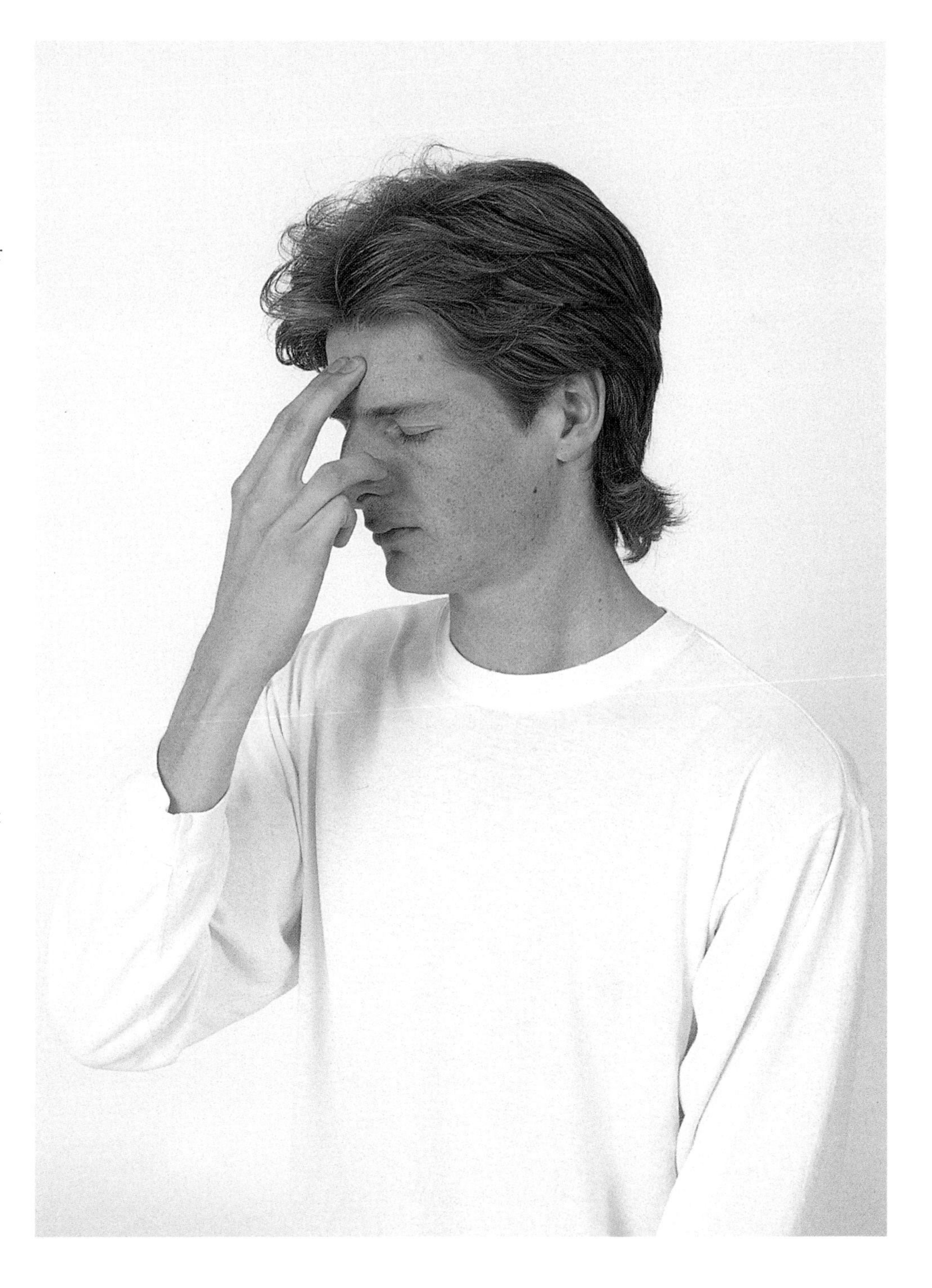

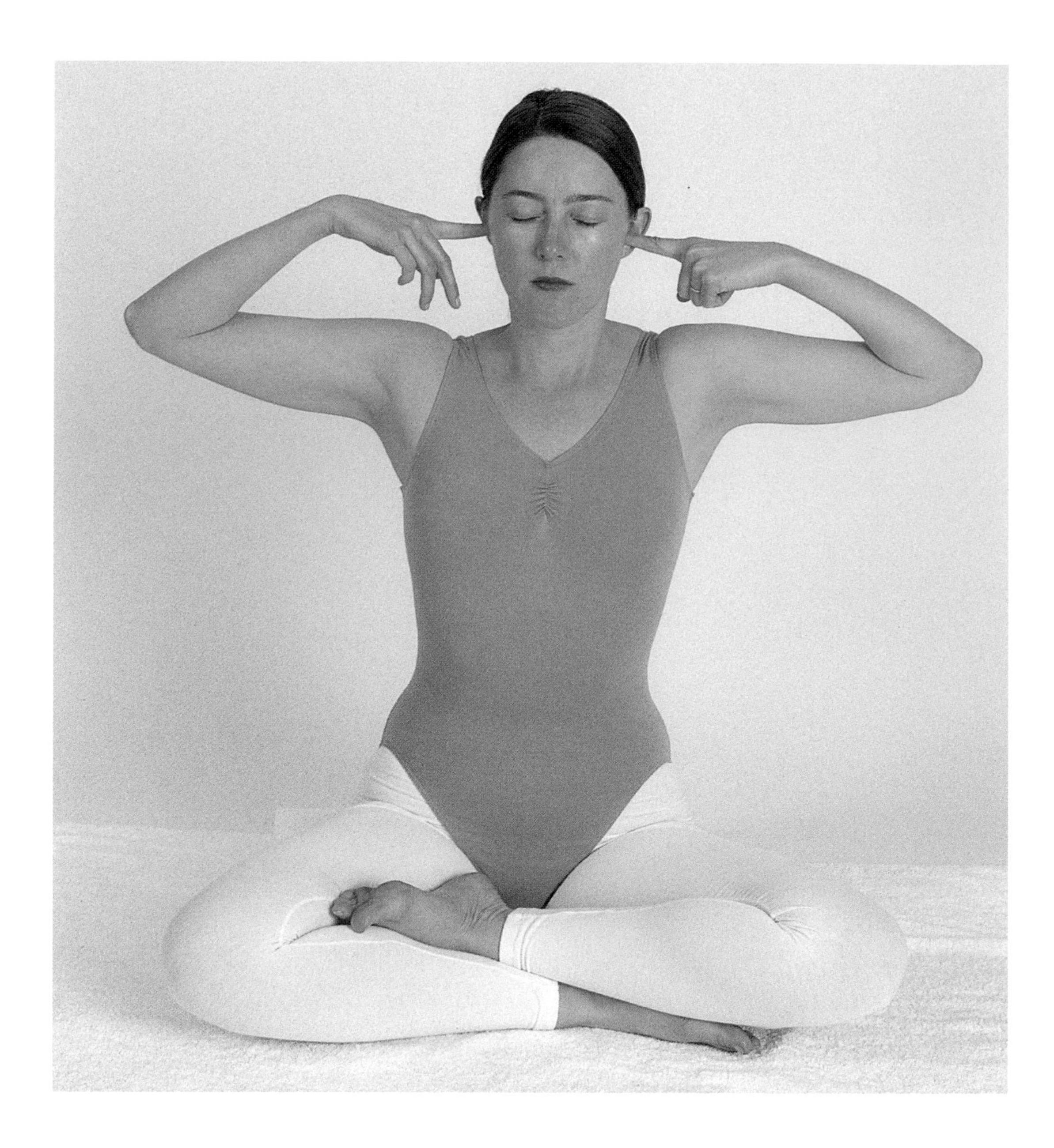

HUMMING BEE BREATH

BHAMARI PRANAYAMA

The Humming Bee Breath is an exhilarating way to clear the mind of excess clutter. Our ability to think clearly is frequently undermined by random thoughts racing around the mind. This exercise quells negative emotions such as anger and anxiety, and helps lower blood pressure. The Humming Bee Breath also strengthens the voice box.

1. Inhale, and place your index fingers in your ears, thus blocking out the noises of the world.

2. As you exhale, make a humming, buzzing sound with your mouth. Keep your mouth closed. Pretend you are a bee. Feel the sound reverberate in the front of your brain. Extend the exhalation as long as you can. Keep your fingers in your ears as you exhale.

3. Repeat the breath several times.

Awareness

Experience the vibration of the sound throughout your mind. Be aware of nothing else.

When you finish the practice, notice how your mind is crisp and lucid. Whenever you feel "frazzled", try the Humming Bee Breath.

Stillness in Meditation

DHYANA

The body is still and the mind is quiet.
Yet you are thoroughly alive, as every cell resounds
with a fresh vitality and comprehension.

To meditate is to create a moment in which there is no time and space is infinite. Daily life is governed by the clock and we all tend to become caught up in our own existence. Through meditation, we gain some refuge from our thoughts and anxieties. This is achieved by learning to control the mind. We create a space of stillness and turn our awareness inwards. By withdrawing from the world, we can return refreshed.

After practicing meditation for some time, you will notice your outlook on life begins to alter. Meditation brings about a subtle change in consciousness. It does not alienate you from the world, but helps you to exist within it with greater happiness.

SOME POINTS TO KEEP IN MIND

- The mind will be better prepared for meditation if preceded by asana and pranayama practices.
- Initially, only meditate for short periods.
- Have no expectations — do not predict what will happen during your meditation. There are no set rules — simply be aware of the process and how it makes you feel. If you experience restlessness, it may be better to leave the practice for that day. Do not be impatient.
- Avoid practicing meditation when you are feeling emotionally unstable, for example, depressed or overly-anxious.

The Chakras

Chakras are "bases" for the body's energy.
The chakras lie along the length of the spine. Each chakra is connected with a different level of existence — for example, instinct, memory, vitality, emotions, creativity, intuition and spirituality. By moving the breath up and down the spine, each of the chakras is activated and balanced.

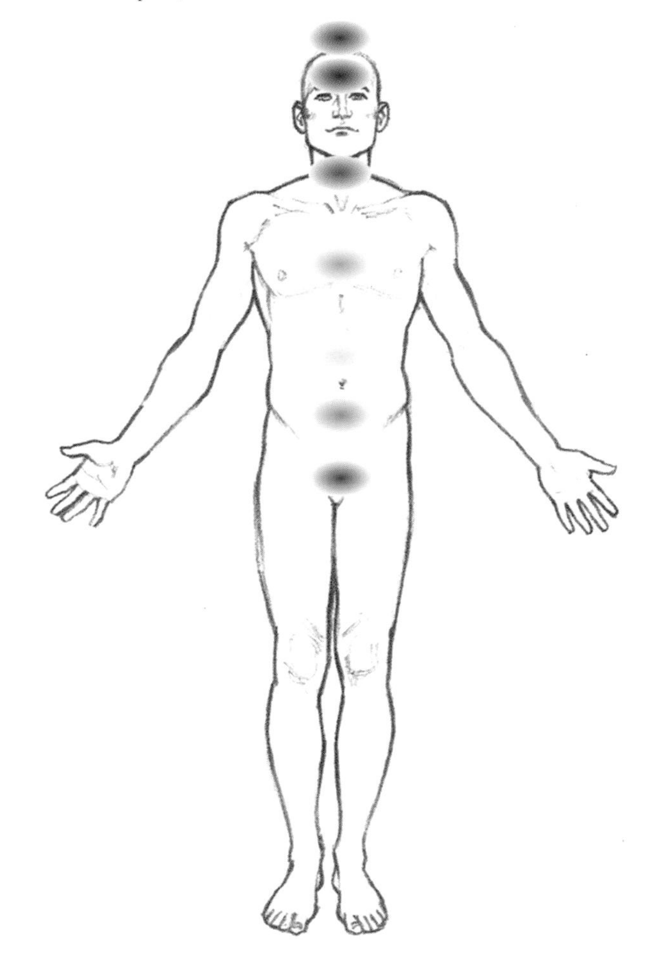

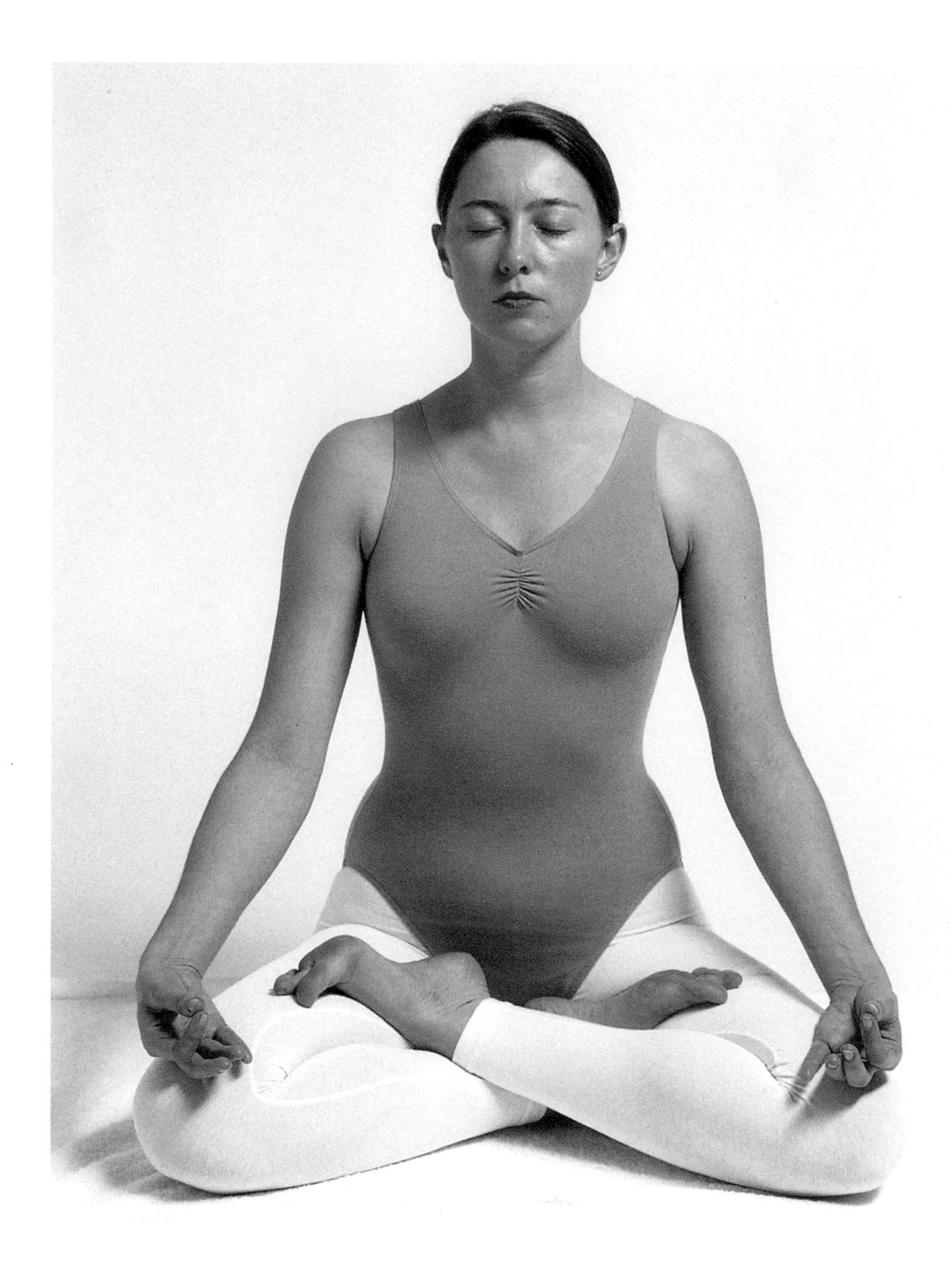

How to Meditate

Even a short meditation can be very beneficial. Try to meditate for just 5 minutes every morning and every night. After your meditation, look around you and notice how your senses have been aroused. It is quite common for colors to look brighter. Sounds may seem clearer and aromas stronger. There are many techniques to explore as you expand your practice. You may like to visualize colors radiating through the body, concentrate on one image or make use of sound such as the "aummm" mantra. The following is a simple meditation practice to begin with.

1. Sit in a comfortable position, as for pranayama — cross-legged, Half-Lotus or Full Lotus (see page 54). Rest your arms on your knees or in your lap. Face palms upwards. If you have just been practicing pranayama, it is best to remain in the same position. Merge one yogic practice into the next.

2. Close your eyes and begin to withdraw your senses from the world. Your body should be straight but relaxed. Remove all tension from the face and neck. Imagine the room in which you are sitting, then let the image disappear.

3. Begin to concentrate on the breath. Observe its passage as it moves in and out. Breathe slowly and fully. As you breathe in, imagine the breath traveling upwards from the base of the spine to the top of the head. As you breathe out, let the breath return to the base of the spine. Now you have stimulated each of the chakras (see page 57).

Notice how you can direct the breath to any part of the body. If you are holding tension somewhere, direct the breath to that point. Release the tension as you breathe out.

4. Now, take your awareness away from the breath, and visualize an infinite space extending from behind your forehead. This space goes on forever. You are no longer conscious of your body. Just enjoy the expanse, and let the mind be still. If thoughts arise, observe them, then let them pass. There is no need to deal with them at this time.

5. Stay in this space for as long as you find it enjoyable.

6. Slowly begin to return to the world. Listen to the sounds around you, imagine the room in which you are sitting once again.

7. When you are ready, open your eyes. Take a moment to make sure you are fully "in" your body and then stretch your legs. If you feel disorientated or simply not ready to move, rest in the Child pose (see page 34).

Total Relaxation

YOGA NIDRA

Every day treat yourself to some time of total rest and relaxation. This process is an essential component of yoga practice.

The ability to achieve a state of total relaxation is one of the most beneficial skills you can possibly learn.

Sitting in an armchair after the day's work may seem like relaxation; but take a moment to observe your body — is it genuinely relaxed? Are you holding tension in your shoulders? Does your back ache? Do thoughts keep racing through your mind?

True relaxation can only come with awareness. The process is simple, but the rewards are vast. By consciously relaxing the body, we expel accumulated stress, calm the mind and restore depleted energy. Overall health is greatly improved. Ideally, practice 5 to 20 minutes of deep relaxation daily. Always include a relaxation in your daily yoga practice. It can be slotted in anywhere in the program – perhaps before beginning the asanas, or before pranayama or after meditation.

How to Relax

Try the following relaxation routines. You may choose to use them all in one session, or concentrate on the one which best suits your needs on the day. There are no rules for relaxation.

1. Letting go

Lie on the floor in the Corpse pose (see page 41). Close your eyes.

Cover yourself with a blanket or light wrap — this will keep you warm and make you feel secure.

Once you have found a comfortable position, inhale, and squeeze every muscle in your body as tightly as possible. Tense the muscles of the face, the arms, the legs, the buttocks. Tighten every bit.

Then with one strong exhalation, release every muscle. Let your body drop onto the floor. Feel the tension being expelled from your body.

Now let your body become very heavy — feel it sink into the floor beneath you.

Lie still and enjoy this sensation. Your body is so heavy, you could not even raise an arm if you tried.

2. Withdrawing the senses

As you lie on the floor, listen to the sounds outside the room. What can you hear in the distance? Observe the sounds — how many different ones can you identify?

Now, leave the sounds outside the room and concentrate on the space around you. Can you hear any noises? Is there a clock ticking? Can you smell anything? Is the temperature hot or cold?

Only be aware of that which surrounds you.

Finally, focus on your own body. Hear your breath moving in and out. Feel the breath. Follow it as it moves in and out of the lungs. Observe the rib cage moving up and down.

Begin to slow the breath down. Fill the body with air. Take two or three full Yogic Breaths (see page 54). The mind and the body is still and quiet. Rest and relax.

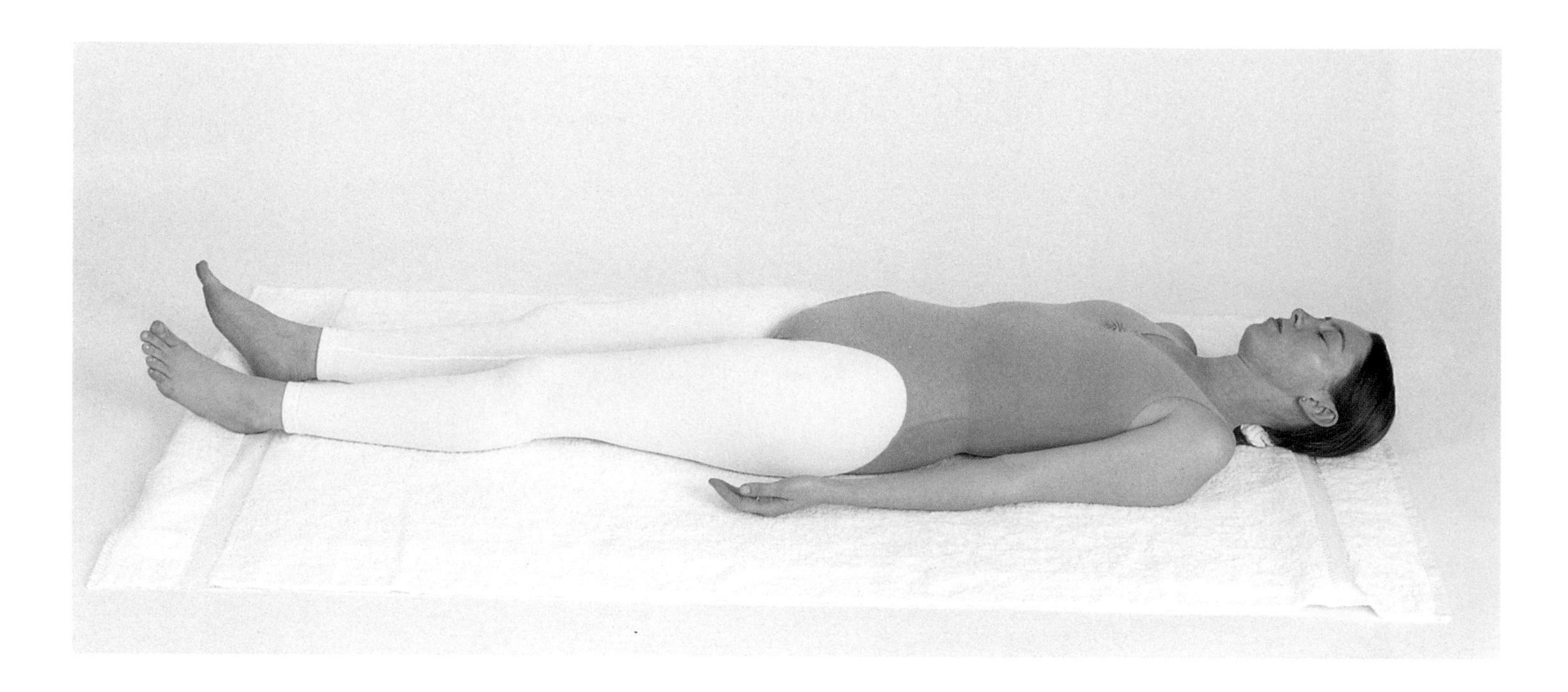

3. Body rotation

Now we will relax each part of the body in turn.

The best way to do this is to name each body part in your mind. As you do so imagine that part relaxing and becoming heavy. Start with the fingers of the right hand.

Whisper in your mind: right thumb... second... third... fourth... little finger... No tension remains in the fingers.

Continue in this manner: the palm of right hand... back of the hand... lower arm... elbow... upper arm... The whole arm is very heavy. The right shoulder... the neck... the head... the right side of the back... the right buttock... the right side of the body...

Now, the right thigh... knee... lower leg... right big toe... second... third... fourth... little toe... all of the right leg...

The whole side of the right body is thoroughly relaxed. Repeat the process on the left side. Release the muscles of the face — the forehead, the eyes, the jaws, the mouth, the nose, the ears. Let go of tightness in the chest and the abdomen. Now the whole body is totally relaxed, the whole body is relaxed and lying on the floor. Say these words to yourself and feel your body respond.

4. Visualization

Another way to relax is to imagine a scene in your mind. Whatever makes you feel happy and calm. You may like to visualize yourself lying in a green field, with the aroma of fresh flowers in the air and the warmth of the sun on your body. A cool stream might flow gently in the background. Listen to it. Perhaps you may like to visualize your body rising above the ground. Now you are looking down at the scene you have created. Let your body float back down to lie in the grass. Your imagination will be your guide.

To help with your body rotation and visualization, try making a tape of the script, and playing it during the relaxation session. This will ease the burden on the mind. Alternatively, you can purchase pre-recorded relaxation tapes at many health and book stores.

5. Return to the world

At the conclusion of the relaxation session, bring your awareness back to the space around you. Feel your body lying on the floor, and imagine the room and all that is in it. Hear the sounds and smell the aromas around you.

Slowly begin to stretch your whole body and then open your eyes.

Rest for a while, before getting up.

Notice how the body and mind feels after a period of total relaxation.

Sequences

The following sequences suggest programs for different times of the day and different situations. Try them out, then create your own practices.

Thirty-minute general sequence

If you can spare half an hour a day, you will benefit from a complete yoga practice. This is one example — there are endless combinations. Once you are familiar with the postures, you can change your practice to suit your mood on each occasion. Try to include:

• Asanas

(you will have time for a short rest between postures)

- warm ups (pages 21-23)	3 minutes
- loosener e.g. Chopping Wood (page 29)	2 minutes
(return to the Mountain rest)	
- balance e.g. Tree (page 26)	2 minutes
(return to the Mountain rest)	
- stretch e.g. Triangle (page 30)	2 minutes
(rest in Forward Bend/Uttanasana, page 25)	
- backward bend e.g. Cobra (page 44)	2 minutes
(rest in Reversed Corpse)	
- forward bend e.g. Dog (page 45)	2 minutes
(rest in the Child)	
- twist (e.g. Half-Spinal Twist, page 40)	2 minutes
• Salute to the Sun (3 rounds) (page 52)	5 minutes
• Corpse pose and relaxation (page 41)	5 minutes
• Pranayama e.g. Alternate Nostril Breath (page 55)	
• a short meditation (page 57)	5 minutes

For the morning

Concentrate on stretching and energizing postures; don't forget pranayama and meditation as these practices make the mind alert for the day's activities.

- Warm ups (pages 21–23)
- Rocking and Rolling (page 42)
- Tree (page 26)
- Cat (page 43)
- Sitting leg stretches — Head to Knee and Wide Leg (page 38)
- Cobra (page 44)
- Triangle (page 30)
- Twisting Triangle (page 32)
- Salute to the Sun — perhaps 1 round slowly, and 2 dynamically (page 52)
- Pranayama — Yogic Breath/Alternate Nostril Breath (pages 54–55)
- Short meditation (page 57)

For the evening

After a day at work, use your yoga practice to restore energy and revitalize the body.

- Wall Stand (page 49)
- Parting of the Clouds (page 28)
- Chopping Wood (page 29)
- Yoga Mudrasana (page 37)
- Infinite Stretch (page 46)
- Dog (page 45)
- Plough or Shoulder Stand (pages 51–50)
- Half-Spinal Twist (page 40)
- Salute to the Sun — gentle rounds (page 52)
- Pranayama — Humming Bee Breath (page 56)
- Meditation (page 57)

Before bedtime

Slow down the body and the mind before retiring to ensure a good night's sleep. Also, it is important to ease the muscles and align the spine before settling down to a long period of rest.

• Warm-ups, especially neck and shoulders (page 21)
• Butterfly (page 35)
• Cat (page 43)
• Cobra (page 44)
• Child (page 34)
• Leg stretches – floor or sitting (pages 38–39, 46)
• Supine Twist (page 47)
• Relaxation (page 59)

Every day

These practices are suitable should you be working in an office, outside in the open air, or at home. As we work, we tend to ignore the stance of our body. Take a break, and "re-connect" from time to time. At the desk occasionally take a break to practice:

• Warm-up exercises – especially neck rolls, shoulder rotation, and shoulder stretch (pages 21–22)

Throughout the day, if you feel your energy flagging and you have the available time and space, try:

• Floppy Twist (page 23)
• Salute to the Sun (page 52)
• Parting of the Clouds (page 28)
• Chopping Wood (page 29)
• Triangle (page 30)
• Twisting Triangle (page 32)

A short pranayama exercise and meditation will help you to maintain concentration during the day.

In the car

While sitting at the traffic lights, ease away tension with:

• Neck Rolls (page 21)
• Shoulder Rotations (page 22)
• Ankle and Wrist Rotations (page 21)
• Yogic Breaths (page 54) – one or two full breaths will relax the body and sharpen the mind. However, do not practice any breathing exercises, except Yogic Breath, while driving!

As you sit in the car, remember to lengthen your spine from the base — this will help prevent backache. After driving, straighten the spine with some twists (pages 40 and 47) , the Triangle (page 30) and the Dog (page 45).

With sport

Before playing any sport or undertaking a strenuous activity, prepare the body with:

• Warm-ups – try them all (pages 21–23)
• Butterfly (page 35)
• Yoga Mudrasana (page 37)
• Looseners: Rocking and Rolling (page 42), Cat (page 43), Chopping Wood (page 29)
• Stretching postures: Head to Knee (page 38), Wide Leg (page 39), Infinite Stretch (page 46)
• Triangle (page 30)
• Salute to the Sun (page 52)

If you wish to enhance your concentration for the activity ahead, try:

• Balances – Tree/Seated Balance (pages 26–36)
• Short pranayama and meditation (pages 54–59)

After sport, soothe and realign the body with:

• More looseners
• More leg stretches
• Twists – Half-Spinal Twist/Supine Twist (pages 40–47)

A relaxation practice is also very therapeutic after sports and exercise.

A stressful event

Try the following postures to tide you through times of stress or high emotion. Before a stressful event try:

• Tree (page 26)
• Cat (page 43)
• Parting of the Clouds (page 28)
• Chopping Wood (page 29)
• Pranayama: Yogic Breath and Alternate Nostril Breath (pages 54–55)
• Meditation practice (page 57)
• Relaxation practice (page 59)

After a stressful event concentrate on these gentle and calming postures:

• Wall Stand (page 49)
• Child (page 34)
• Supine Twist (page 47)
• Plough (page 51)
• Shoulder Stand (page 50)
• Pranayama: Yogic Breath and Humming Bee Breath (pages 54–56)
• Relaxation practice (page 59)

For menstruation

The most appropriate postures to practice during menstruation, are:

- Butterfly (page 35)
- Supine Butterfly (Supta Baddha Konasana) — from the Butterfly position, gently lower the back onto the floor (see photo, opposite) — this position is very soothing during menstruation.
- Cat (page 43)
- Sitting stretches: Head to Knee and Wide Leg (pages 38 and 39)
- Relaxation – lying in the Corpse pose, and practicing slow Yogic Breaths is also very beneficial should you be experiencing any discomfort or stress.

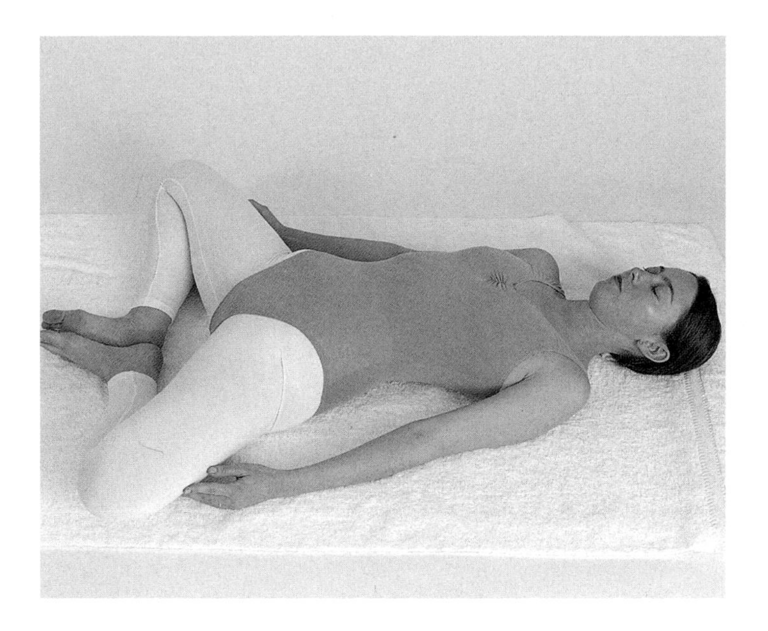

Yoga and the Rest of Your Life

At the close of this book, you will have an insight into the total practice of yoga. The postures, the breathing, the meditation and the relaxation are all simple and gentle exercises. Yet they work strongly on body, mind and energy to bring harmony to your existence.

The body becomes toned, the mind sharp and the emotions calm. Overall health is significantly improved.

Now that you understand the basis of yoga, incorporate it into your daily life. You will soon notice a difference in the way you stand, sit, move, think and feel.

Developing the ability to have some control over your body, mind and your essential energy is the unique gift of yoga. If you enjoy the practice, let yoga be your friend and helper as you travel through your lifetime.

First published in Great Britain in 1996
by Chancellor Press
a division of Reed Consumer Books
Michelin House, 81 Fulham Rd, London SW3 6RB

Published in conjunction with Lansdowne Publishing Pty Ltd
Level 5, 70 George Street, Sydney, NSW 2000, Australia

Set in Caslon 540 Roman on Quark Xpress
Printed in Singapore by Tien Wah Press (Pte) Ltd

National Library of Australia Cataloguing-in-Publication data

Bailey, Karen, 1963 –
The gentle art of yoga: a step-by-step to easy exercises at home.
ISBN 1 85152 918 7
I. Yoga. I. Title
613.7046

Page 8: The visit of a Prince to an Ascetic, c.1830, Indian
Oriental Museum, Durham University/Bridgeman Art Library, London